Your child

from birth

to eight

3rd edition

D1725875

Pam Linke

ACER Press

This third edition published 2012
by ACER Press, an imprint of
Australian Council for Educational Research Ltd
19 Prospect Hill Road, Camberwell
Victoria, 3124, Australia

www.acerpress.com.au
sales@acer.edu.au

Second edition published 1996
First edition published 1989

Edited by Maureen O'Keefe
Cover design, text design and typesetting by ACER Project Publishing
Cover image: © Vanessa Nel/Shutterstock.com
Printed in Australia by BPA Print Group

p.135: *The Very Hungry Caterpillar* by Eric Carle. Used by permission of
Penguin Group (USA) Inc. All rights reserved.

National Library of Australia Cataloguing-in-Publication entry:
Author: Linke, Pam.
Title: Your child from birth to eight / Pam Linke.
Edition: 3rd ed.
ISBN: 9781742860282 (pbk.)
Notes: Includes index.
Subjects: Child development.
Dewey Number: 305.231

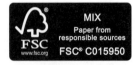

Foreword

If only a book with this much clarity and wisdom, based as it is upon decades of scientific research and professional experience, could be made widely available to all new parents. There is pure gold in these pages: just the kind of treasure (information, understanding, sharing) that all parents require in the process of seeking to nurture their children.

The life of infants and young children is simply too important to go without the wise counsel of wise teachers. Pam Linke, with her more than 30 years of knowledge focusing on the all-important and specific needs of children, has done us all a remarkable favour. She has distilled into this wonderful book so much of what is required for provision of genuine security in our children. She is to be commended and parents are to be congratulated each time they turn to these pages.

Dr. Kent Hoffman
Infant, Child and Adult Psychotherapy
Co-originator of Circle of Security®
Washington, United States

For my grandchildren
Scarlett, Charlie, Leo and Gabriella
who are giving me a whole new
experience of young children's development
and who bring such joy to our family.

Contents

Acknowledgements

I would like to acknowledge Peter Bowler who wrote the first edition of *Your child from one to ten*, which I revised and updated for the second edition. Writing a book to give parents information about the ages and stages that their children pass through was Peter's idea and, while this is a completely new edition with added sections on parenting, the basic structure is based, with permission, on his original edition.

I would like to thank the parents and children whose photographs are used in this book.

I would also like to thank Dr Elizabeth Puddy, Dr Christy Ward, Sue Higgins and Andrea McGuffog for helpful comments and constructive criticism. Any mistakes are mine, but the text is improved by their wisdom. I would also like to thank my husband who has allowed me the time to work on this book and done more than his share of babysitting grandchildren.

Finally, I would like to acknowledge my work colleagues, and especially my own children and grandchildren who have taught me much – I am still learning.

Introduction

Your child from birth to eight is about how young children grow and learn and how parents, carers and educators can promote children's development. While young children generally go through more or less the same developmental steps, particularly within the same community and culture, what and how they learn is very much influenced by their environment, the people they are close to and the way they are parented and taught. For example, generally 2-year-olds may climb up and down stairs but a child who has lived with stairs is likely to do it at a much younger age than a child who has never seen stairs. Knowing your own child and how he or she is growing and learning is the key. Use this book as a guide, to help you understand more about how children generally grow and develop and to give you ideas about helping your child build the skills and strengths he or she needs. It may also help you to know if your child is very out-of-step in any way with others of the same age.

This book is a third edition – the second edition was published as *Your child from one to ten*. Since the publication of *Your child from one to ten* there has been an explosion of knowledge about young children, and what influences their learning and development. New research highlights the importance of children's earliest years and how parents and carers can help them to get the best start in their lives; due to this research there are many changes in this third edition. At the same time, this book includes fundamental information that has not changed over the years.

Another change to this edition is that the age range is birth to 8. This is because it is in a baby's first year that the foundations for the future are built. By the age of 3 your baby's brain has done most of its growing and pathways that link the cells in the brain have been laid down.[1] Early experiences have the biggest impact on how the brain develops, although learning and development continue throughout life. The book finishes at the age of 8 because the years from birth to 8 are critically important to children's development. In Australia and internationally (including UNESCO[2]) these are considered the early years, when children develop and learn most rapidly. This is when parenting is crucially important and this book is intended to support parents as you help your child along the path to a happy and successful life.

There is a chapter for each year from birth to 8, covering general developmental expectations, the things that influence children, and suggestions for you to support your child's learning and development. Many of these suggestions come from the wisdom of parents and educators with whom I have worked over the years, together with current knowledge about children.

Some of the information about social behaviour, for example that four-year-olds can be boisterous is, of course, a generalisation. Many four-year-olds do behave in this way. Many children, however, due to their own temperament and life experiences, are very different. As long as your child is happy and gets on well with other people it is nothing to worry about. It takes all kinds of people to make a world.

There is extra information in each chapter that is relevant for children of that age, and sometimes other ages as well – some things that you might wish someone had told you before your child reached that age.

Many fathers take equal responsibility with mothers in caring for babies nowadays, so in some ways it seems unnecessary to have dedicated sections for fathers. However, many dads were brought up in families where parental roles were very separate so the fathers' sections are provided as a guide for those who want it.

Parenting is the most important predictor of children's outcomes. The most supportive parenting involves love, positive communication, appropriate limits, monitoring where your children are and what they are doing, positive discipline and spending time with them. This is both a responsibility and a wonderful opportunity.

The best way to support children's development is to love them and to provide opportunities to play and explore and learn, use positive discipline and ensure safe limits for them. Talk and listen, watch and play with your child, and think about how this amazing new being is taking on the huge and exciting task of making sense of, adapting to and making his or her way in the world.

No parent is perfect and children learn much about relationships from mistakes and reconnections. This book is meant to reassure and support parents and families. I wish you well and hope that the information provided here will be helpful to you as you love, care for and guide your children.

> **Note:** In this book 'he' and 'she' are used alternately in different chapters when talking about a child. Unless it specifically says differently 'he' and 'she' refer to both sexes.

Guide to using this book

Each chapter is divided into sections about physical, social/emotional, speech and language development, as well as thinking and learning, followed by other topics that parents often want to know about. In fact all of these things overlap as young children's learning takes place in a holistic way. So when your baby, for example, looks at a picture book on your lap she is learning:

▶ about language and how words tell stories
▶ that books are important because the person she loves best enjoys them
▶ to feel safe and secure and loved in her parent's arms.

All of these combine to contribute to her future as a reader.

At the end of each chapter is a brief summary of the development in that year, and a list of suitable toys or gifts. These are general suggestions, to use if they fit your child. All children are individual and develop in their own way and time.

At the back of the book, under the heading 'References' is a list of the books that have been referred to throughout the text (a reference is indicated by a superscript number).

Because this book has a broad scope, there will probably be some topics where you will want more information. On pages 192–96 are some suggestions of books and websites which will be interesting and helpful for further reading or research, including some for children.

This book refers to mothers and fathers and I would like to acknowledge the many families who have different structures such as stepfamilies, gay families, adoptive families and single parent households, and the many other people who care for children but are not their birth parents. The book is about how children grow and develop and how best to support their development, whatever your role in caring for or educating them. Where mothers or fathers are mentioned it will usually be possible to adapt the information to your own situation.

One very important aspect for children is that the adults who care for them every day love them and love each other, or at least care about and treat each other with respect. This is the foundation for children to thrive. Without it their development and wellbeing is likely to be compromised. If parenting or family relationships are not working well for you, if you feel uncomfortable about something or your child is not doing as well as you would like, you need to get help for the sake of your child.

Key topics across the age range

Some topics appear in specific chapters although they may apply across the age range. These include:

Attention seeking (p. 110)

Bedwetting (p. 109)

Bullying (p. 139)

Child care (p. 35)

Computers (p. 88)

Discipline (p. 43, 86, 107, 181)

Family breakup (p. 23)

Laughing (p. 85)

Managing feelings (p. 34)

Motivation (p. 180)

New baby (p. 65)

Optimism (p. 149)

Play (p. 104)

Play-based learning (p. 105)

Problem solving (p. 142)

Resilience (p. 89)

Sibling rivalry (p. 129)

Spirituality (p. 92)

Superhero play (p. 109)

Tantrums (p. 55)

Temperament (p. 67)

Values (p. 165)

Children's needs

A number of child development experts over the years[3,4] have made recommendations for what children need in order to have the best opportunities for development, wellbeing, health and happiness.

Below is a summary of this research:

▶ Physical needs – food, sleep, warmth, shelter, health care, safety (including safety from emotional and physical abuse in their home, either towards the child or between parents).

▶ Love and security – children need to know there are people they can rely on to love them and care for them and provide predictability in their lives; for example, be there when they say they will be, provide comfort in times of stress, give support to try new things.

▶ Opportunities to experiment and explore and learn – opportunities for mastery, skill building, persistence building, exercise/physical health and encouragement in their endeavours.

▶ Positive discipline – setting boundaries for and with children, positive communication and knowing where children are and what they are doing. Positive discipline sees misbehaviour as something a child needs help with, rather than requiring punishment.

▶ Caring environments – children know where they belong and that there are people around them who support them (cultural groups, early childhood services and school, people who support their parents, and safe neighbourhoods)

▶ Parents and carers who enjoy their children and have fun with them.

Chapter 1
Birth to One – the first year

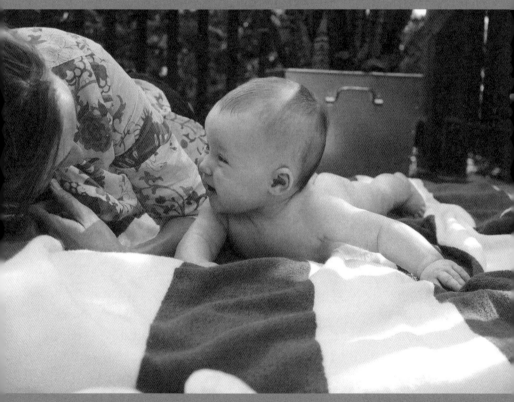

Getting to know your baby

The first year of your baby's life is an amazing journey for both parents and baby. Newborn babies seem very helpless. Yet even from birth they can cry to get help when they are hungry or uncomfortable, suck when they need to feed, make eye contact with you to start building relationships, and relax when they are contented. In the first year they will be able to roll over, sit up, crawl, and perhaps be taking their first steps. They hold things in their hands, manipulate toys, and may say some words. They are social members of the family and they learn this from the start.

Physical development

New babies cannot yet regulate all of their body functions; for example, they need you to make sure they are not too hot or too cold. Keeping their heads uncovered when they are sleeping indoors helps them not get too hot. If you feel comfortable with the temperature and the clothing you are wearing, your baby is probably OK in similar clothes.

At first, many of your baby's movements are reflex. The movements just happen and the baby has no control over them, such as throwing out her arms when something startles her. In a very few days after birth you will see your baby start to turn her head when lying on her back. However, newborn babies don't have strong neck muscles and they need you to support their heads when you hold them in the early weeks. By 2 months your baby will be able to lift her head when lying on her tummy, and over the next month or two she will learn to prop herself up on her arms. By 3 to 4 months she will try to hit or kick a toy within reach and, especially if it makes a noise, she will continue to practise until she has learned to control this new movement. During this time her muscles are getting stronger, readying her for crawling and walking.

Babies usually don't sleep on their tummies because of the risk of Sudden Infant Death Syndrome (SIDS) <www.sidsandkids.org>. They need daytime play on their tummies, with supervision from an adult, beginning from the first weeks. Tummy time strengthens the muscles they use for controlling their heads, sitting up, crawling and walking. Some babies don't like being on their tummy, except in the bath. You can help your baby to enjoy it by sitting on the floor and letting her lie over your knees or lying on the floor and letting her lie over your tummy. Try putting some interesting toys in front of her, or lying on the floor yourself and facing her, while singing or talking to her.

Your baby enjoys kicking her legs and waving her arms about – getting lots of exercise ready for purposeful movement. She needs to kick and play on the floor without too many clothes to restrict her movement. Put some things that she likes to look at within her reach to encourage her to reach out. Hold her upright, while gently supporting her head at first, to give her practice at controlling her head. Make it an opportunity to talk, sing and smile with her.

By about 3 months she holds her hands together much of the time, rather than have one arm out and the other bent. She is getting her eyes and hands to work together, and managing to hit a rattle when she wants to and to hold one for a short time. Between 4 and 6 months your baby will start to roll over from back to front and back again to her great delight.

She will enjoy finding her hands and feet and spend much time looking at them, even managing to get her feet into her mouth. She puts most things in her mouth when she can; this is one way she learns so keep small things out of her reach to avoid choking. By 5 to 6 months she can move around a lot, probably not crawling, but pivoting around on the floor when she is on her tummy. By now she has better head control and can help hold her head steady when you pull her up to sitting.

Between 6 and 12 months, she works on holding things such as a spoon or small block and passing them from one hand to the other. As she gets better at using her hands, she will pick up small objects such as a pea or try pulling the hairs on your arms with her thumb and finger. She will also try to get hold of your hair or glasses or jewellery.

By 7 to 8 months most babies can sit up with straight backs, although they are a bit precarious at first and may need a cushion behind them in case they topple over. In the last part of the first year your baby will learn to go from sitting to lying on the floor and back to sitting again. Placing toys within reach alongside as well as in front of them helps babies to learn to turn their bodies and be more flexible. They start to crawl any time after the age of 6 months, although a few babies don't crawl 'properly' at all but hitch themselves around on their bottoms or do a commando-type crawl on their tummies. Many babies crawl backwards before they go forwards. Once they are crawling well they may crawl on hands and feet to avoid scraping their knees on the floor.

By 9 months your baby will probably pull herself up to standing and walk around furniture. For some babies it can take weeks or even months after this to learn to balance well enough to take that first step. Other babies seem to do it within a few days of standing. Once she gets onto her feet your baby will enjoy practising walking, either holding your hand or pushing a toy on wheels. (Make sure that the toy is heavy enough not to run away from her.) There is a wide age difference between when babies learn to walk, some as young as 9 months and others 15 months or older.

> Four-month-old Gabby has just learned to roll from her back to her tummy. She is so excited by her new skill that she cannot stop doing it: as soon as she is put on her back she rolls over again. The first night after this development, when she woke for a feed, she would not stay on her back and spent much of the night being put on her back and rolling over again straight away. Fortunately, after a couple of nights she seemed to feel that she did not need to do it all the time and went back to her usual sleeping habits.
>
> *Achieving skills is very exciting for babies. Once they have really mastered them they move on to something new.*

Seeing and hearing

When babies are born they can't see far very clearly and sometimes their eyes don't seem to work well together. They see best at about 30 to 40 centimetres, just the right distance to watch their parent's face when held in the arms for feeding. Looking at your baby when she looks at you, gazing into each other's eyes, helps her learn about who you are and that you are there to care for her. Watch for your baby's response when you show her things. If she likes to look she will go on looking; if the thing is too close or too far away, or she does not like it, she will squirm or turn her head or maybe shut her eyes. By 6 months she is able to see fairly well and look at things and people across the room and further away.

From birth babies can hear well and like to listen to your voice. At first they startle at loud noises, but household noises don't usually wake them if they are asleep. In fact, gentle noise in the background can help them sleep while complete silence may make it harder. It is not quiet in the uterus before they are born and that is what they are used to.

From the start your baby will enjoy listening to your voice as you talk about what you are doing. Her listening is the beginning of her learning to talk as well as getting to know you.

Social and emotional development

Your baby starts to recognise you from birth – your voice, your touch, your smell and how you look. By the end of the first 3 months she can turn her head and listen when she hears your voice. She follows your movements with her eyes. Babies smile after the first few weeks and by 3 or 4 months become very sociable, laughing and gurgling and smiling at anyone who comes by. Although she is learning to know you, your baby still doesn't understand that you are separate from her and she sees you come and go as if by magic.

During the early months your baby needs you to respond as soon as possible when she is upset, hungry or frightened and to be gentle and warm and give her lots of smiles and loving touch. Even very new babies look at the face of the person who is feeding or talking to them. Young babies who are upset are calmer when they are held by someone they are used to.

Young babies need to learn about the world slowly and gently, a bit at a time. Too many new experiences or lots of people holding them can make them distressed. Babies show they are feeling stressed in other ways besides crying – such as looking away, looking upset, yawning, hiccups, arching back and even going to sleep.[5]

Babies build up a picture of the world during this time. They first need to develop trust that they are safe and cared for and that someone will come when they are hungry, afraid, lonely or just needing love. This trust develops over the first few months of life and it happens because you are reliable, you come when she cries, you hold her when she is sad, you feed her when she is hungry and you delight in her. Babies and children who have this kind of start in life expect other people to be friendly and they are friendly themselves. When they learn to trust others and get along well with people it stands them in good stead in their future lives. When a person has friends and close, supportive relationships, it makes learning easier, getting and keeping a job easier and coping with troubles easier. And the foundations for all this are laid down in the first year of life!

The best way you can help is by responding to your baby's cues, gently playing with her, and being predictable (so she knows what to expect) and loving. Help your baby learn what to expect by telling her what you are going to do with her in the same words each time, for example: 'Now I am going to pick you up'; 'Now I am changing your nappy'. This helps her to feel secure and builds confidence, even though she doesn't understand the words. It would be scary even for an adult if they never knew what to expect from the person they were closest to.

By about 6 or 7 months (see **Thinking and Learning**) your baby realises that her parents, who are the most important people in her world, come and go and she might now be frightened or worried when you go. This is sometimes called separation anxiety and is a normal part of learning and growing. A baby who went to sleep easily a few weeks ago may now need you to comfort her at bedtime. Your friendly, sociable baby may be afraid of other people, even people she knows quite well. Crawling babies try to follow you as you move about the house. Your baby ventures a little way away from you and then comes back, or perhaps just looks back to be sure you are still there. Separation anxiety is likely to last for many months, as she learns to deal with her new expanding world. Although it gradually diminishes, for most children it is not until they are about 3 that they usually cope well with longer separations from their main carer(s). If you know that this is normal and meet your baby's needs without being worried yourself or annoyed at her clinging, she will gradually get her inner confidence and be able to do more and more on her own.

There will be times when you have to leave your child for a while when she doesn't want you to. Leave her with someone she knows well and trusts if you can, and make sure you say 'Good-bye' and let her know when you will be back. She does not understand the words fully but your reassuring tone helps build her trust. It is tempting to sneak out so she won't be upset, but this makes babies worry because they never know whether you will be there or not. Let her know you understand she is upset but you will soon be back and you are not worried. Young children learn much about what is safe in the world from your attitude. If you aren't scared of something, your children are less likely to be.

When babies are stressed, such as being exposed to parents' anger or often being left to cry, their brains develop sensitivity to stress which interferes with their learning in all other areas. Babies can be stressed by too little attention, where the adults in their lives are too busy to respond to them. They can also be stressed by adults who try too hard to help, so the babies don't get space to try things out for themselves and/or the time to explore one thing properly before moving on to something else. The way to work this out is to watch your baby and notice when she wants more interaction and when she needs a break, and to follow her cues.

Baby cues

Learning to know what your baby's signs and signals (cues) mean and responding to them is one of the most important parts of being a parent.

Every baby has their own particular way of showing you what they need but there are some signs you can watch out for. Babies who want to play or 'talk' with you look alert and interested. Babies who need a change or are unhappy may yawn, look away, grizzle, grimace or even go to sleep. Tired babies may grizzle or yawn or get agitated. You help your baby best when you learn what her cues mean and respond to them, but this takes time. Even when you don't understand what your baby needs (and this happens often at first), your baby knows that you are there caring for her, and this is what matters.

Your baby loves you to play little games with her, but watch for her signals about what she likes and when she has had enough. Some games such as giggling and tickling games are too overwhelming for young babies and are best kept for when they are older.

Speech and language

Babies are born with the ability to speak all languages. Over the first year, as you speak to your baby in your own language, the ability to make some of the sounds of other languages disappears.[6] Your baby learns language from the time she is born, by listening to you as you talk and sing with her. When she makes her own little noises stop and show you are listening and then copy them back to her. Wait for her to make another attempt so she knows you are hearing her and making space for her to 'talk'. Then again copy what she says. This says to her that you have heard what she is saying and you are interested in her early conversations. You can also show interest and interact with her by copying her gestures as well, so if she pokes her tongue out for example, you can do it back and then wait for her to have another go. This is practising the turn-taking patterns we use in conversation. Remember to watch for signals that she wants to talk with you (looking alert and smiling) or she has had enough (looking away, wriggling around, grizzling).

As you say the names of things repeatedly, and her own name of course, she is starting to learn her first words. You can teach language best by fitting words with actions so your baby sees you do something as you say it. She also may enjoy copying you as you make the sounds, for example of a fish or blow raspberries. Your baby may like to copy you as you touch and name parts of your body and her body, such as nose, eyes, ears, tummy and feet, and enjoy making a game of it.

In the last three or four months of her first year, she may start to make meaningful words. At first she just makes sounds such as 'mm-m' which seems like 'mum, mum', especially to mothers! When you show delight as she does this, it encourages her to experiment further and to start to link it to the word 'mum'. Even at this young age they understand a lot of what you are saying to them, long before they can say the words themselves. They can also make hand signs and use them to communicate. Some parents teach their babies sign language to aid communication before speech – simple signs such as 'milk', 'more' and 'sleep' can help you understand your baby's needs. Signing may help language develop and it also enables babies to feel understood.[7] One-year-olds sometimes make up their own signs as well.

Babies may wave 'bye-bye' or blow a kiss when you ask them to and start to obey simple sentences such as 'Show me the book' or 'Give me the spoon'.

You help your baby learn to talk by spending lots of time talking to her and also reading books to her, beginning from the first few weeks. Start with books that have clear pictures of things she knows, name them for her and/or make their sounds. Babies especially like to look at faces and very clear patterns, as well as both bright colours and black and white.

By the end of the first year you will be starting to say 'no' sometimes as she crawls towards something that might hurt her. She learns what it means as you say it and move her away at the same time. She may start to obey it sometimes, but don't expect her to catch on quickly.

All this is the beginning of literacy that is so important to everything we do.

Thinking and learning

One of the most important developments in research is knowledge about how babies' brains develop. The brain is the only body organ that is not complete at birth. When your baby is born the brain structure is there, but many important linkages between the brain cells are developed with usage after birth. In the next

Neuroscience

Neuroscience is the study of the brain and the nervous system. Over recent years there has been a huge amount of research into what happens to the brain before birth and in infancy and how that affects children's development. This has shown that what happens in the first weeks, months and years of life is crucial to how children's brains develop. Combined with other sciences such as psychology, anthropology and medicine, there has also been a lot of research about what parents and carers can do to provide the best conditions to support brain development and provide the best outcomes for children.[8,9]

few years the brain will grow millions of cells and connections between these cells that are the foundation for everything that your baby's brain will be able to do in the future. What you do with your baby in the first years, especially the first year, is actually helping to develop her brain. If she has good experiences about learning new things, encouragement when she needs it and lots of opportunities to explore, the connections for thinking and learning will be strengthened. Most of all, loving care and lots of gentle loving touch are important for brain development. Over time those connections in the brain that are used less can become weaker and ones that aren't used at all may disappear. Taking care of your baby's brain development is one of your most important responsibilities.

One of the big learning steps of the first year comes at about 6 or 7 months when babies learn that things exist when they can't see them. Before this it is literally out of sight out of mind.

Object permanence

A pioneer researcher into child development, Jean Piaget, developed the idea of object permanence to explain why young babies don't look for something once it goes out of their sight. Young babies don't realise that an object can still exist if they can't see, hear or touch it. For the same reason young babies also don't get upset when their mother goes out of the room. At some stage babies show that they know hidden objects still exist. They may practise this new knowledge by dropping a spoon from their high chair, looking over the chair and seeing it, then wanting you to pick it up so they can drop it again. Early scientific experimenting! Or a baby may pull a blanket over her face and then pull it down to check that you are still there. And they love to play peek-a-boo as they work out that you will still be there each time. Piaget thought that this development occurs at about 7–8 months but current researchers have shown that it sometimes happens much earlier.[10]

The secrets with thinking and learning in the first year are to:

- make sure that your baby feels loved and secure so she is relaxed and open to learning
- give your baby lots of gentle touching and holding
- give your baby different things to look at and do – for example walks in the pram, keeping her with you as you work, and different things to touch and hold
- read, sing and talk to your baby a lot
- let your baby learn at her own pace and follow her lead about what she wants to do, encouraging her when she is having a go. Give her a change or a rest when she has had enough. This gives her the best chance to learn.

Remember that babies learn about things by putting them in their mouths so keep small objects away from them.

> Leo was in his mother's arms as she unlocked the door. He showed that he wanted the key. She put down her shopping and gave it to him but he could not get the key into the lock. She gently turned the key over and he successfully got it in. He chuckled with delight at his new achievement.
>
> *Encouraging children to try things without taking over assists them to develop a sense of self-efficacy.*

Play

Babies love to play. They play with their own fingers and toes. They play with toys that make a noise or move when they touch them and they respond to bright colours. They love to play cuddling games with parents and have parents blow raspberries on their tummies. From 6 months onwards they enjoy peek-a-boo games. They love you to dance and sing with them (including singing about what you are doing) and show them picture books every day. They enjoy finger plays and rhymes. Play is how babies learn. Practising with toys and play helps them to move forward in their development.

Sleeping

Most parents hope that their babies will sleep well, but in fact it is rare for parents of babies not to be tired, at least some of the time. Young babies sleep a lot, just waking for feeds and a few short wake times, including waking several times at night. When they are very young they need regular feeds across the 24 hours.

There are two reasons for this. One reason is nutrition. Breastfeeding, where possible, is best for babies and breast milk is made so babies can digest it easily and quickly which means they are soon hungry again. Secondly, babies' sleep cycles are shorter than adults' and they go into lighter sleep or stir after about 40 to 45 minutes. This is an opportunity to be ready to re-settle them before they fully wake (if they do not need a feed).

By about 3 months, sometimes sooner, babies learn to sleep longer at night and may go five hours at a stretch. This is considered 'sleeping through' for babies. How well babies sleep depends on a number of things, including temperament, noise, how you settle the baby to sleep, developmental and emotional issues and cultural sleeping practices. Breastfed babies are likely to wake more often for feeds. When they reach about 6 or 7 months, even previously good sleepers may start to be anxious at bedtime or wake at night and need some parental comforting, due to separation anxiety. In time they are able to hold in their minds the knowledge that you are there to comfort them if they need it and so go back to sleep on their own. This varies with different babies and takes time.

There are different ways to settle babies to sleep and many people have strong opinions on these. Some people sleep near or with their babies (sleeping in the same room as your baby is recommended by many health professionals for the first year as it seems to be a protection against sudden infant death). Others have their babies in a separate room or sharing a room with another child. If you think about what helps adults to sleep it might help you with ideas for settling your baby. This might include:

- feeling physically comfortable at bedtime – not hungry or thirsty or too hot or too cold

- having a bedtime routine – for example warm bath, soft music, reading a book
- feeling emotionally comfortable – not upset, frightened, angry, stressed, lonely.

If you think about these things in relation to your baby you will be well on the way to helping her sleep, remembering that babies need feeds more often, have shorter sleep cycles and have a lot less understanding of the world than older children. Whatever method and place you choose for your baby to sleep, the important things are to know that your baby is safe both physically and emotionally. You can check safe sleep guidelines on the SIDS website <www.sidsandkids.org>.

Babies learn to feel secure in the world by being responded to when they cry, so the time parents put in to responding to and comforting their babies is very worthwhile. Putting your baby's cot right alongside your bed enables you to respond quickly to her needs.

Eating

Between 4 and 6 months babies start taking an interest in food and may be ready to try solid foods. At first they are likely to push their food straight out again, not because they don't like it but because it takes time to work out how to manage their tongues to keep it in and swallow. If your baby doesn't seem to like a particular food, wait a few days and try again. Feeding needs to be something she enjoys and babies and children do best if they don't feel pressured. Babies learning to eat are often messy as they learn about food by putting their hands in it and trying to feed themselves. Putting newspaper under the highchair is one way of allowing your child to explore this new part of her life while keeping your own cool.

Some other things to know about babies

Attachment

Attachment has different meanings. Nursing mothers talk about the importance of good attachment to the breast for example (see below). Attachment in this section means how secure does the baby feel with her parent or main caregiver. The original understanding of attachment came from a researcher called John Bowlby. He worked out that babies seem to have one main person whom they feel safest with and that this safe feeling is the foundation for future relationships and confidence, a kind of map for how they expect the world to be for them. When babies have a secure attachment it means that they feel secure, so they learn to be friendly and willing to have a go at things. Bowlby's theory[11] emerged from observing the need of infants to be protected and cared for; as infants learn that there is someone who provides this protection and care, this person becomes very important to them. Babies can have more than one attachment person but usually one person is most important when they are young.

> 'There is abundant evidence that almost every child habitually prefers one person, usually his mother-figure, to whom to go when distressed, but that, in her absence he will make do with someone else, preferably someone whom he knows well. On these occasions most children show a clear hierarchy of preference...'[12]

Attachment involves:

- the special person being **a secure base** to explore the world from and to come back to for reassurance. Babies act as if they are on an elastic apron string: they move out, then come back to 'check in', then move out a bit further as they gain more confidence. Gradually, by the time they are about 3, they can spend and enjoy longer periods away from their attachment person or people without being stressed, because they have inner confidence about themselves and others.

• the special person being a **safe haven** to come back to when they are stressed and need comfort. When they get the comfort they need they feel OK to move out again to do things by themselves.

Attachment cycle. The cycle of attachment involves the child being with their parent (secure base) → moving out to explore or play → feeling insecure, unsure → returning to the parent for comfort → receiving comfort and returning to play →

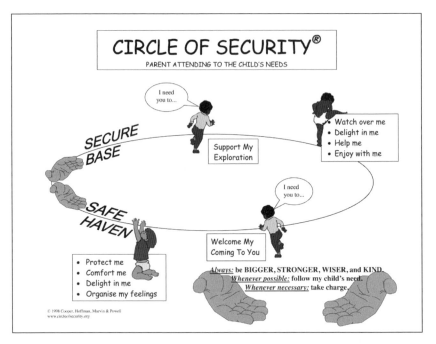

Figure 1.1   Circle of Security diagram[13]   *Source: www.circleofsecurity.net*

How parents can help

Parents help by being available when the child needs comfort, supporting their exploration and welcoming their return. When the attachment needs are strongest, often from about 7 months to about 2 years, it can be wearing for parents as babies may become very clingy, have a greater need for support at bedtime, and may not want to go with other people, sometimes even people they know well. It helps to remind yourself that this is normal and that the best way to get through it is to respond to the child's needs without being either anxious or irritated. A secure attachment is a very positive basis for a child's future development. As your baby feels more secure she will be gradually more willing to be apart from you for longer periods of time.

If your child is sad when you leave, make sure you spend some time when you come back to reconnect with her and reinforce the safe haven part of the attachment cycle (see Figure 1.1).

Attachment to the breast

Breastfeeding is the best way to feed babies and most mothers want to do it successfully. However, with first babies it is often harder at first than you expect and it can hurt until your breasts get used to it. If you understand that this is normal and persevere through the first few weeks, most mothers find that it is satisfying and rewarding as well as good for your baby. Support from an understanding lactation consultant or lactation-trained maternal child health nurse can be invaluable. If you are unable to breastfeed, your baby will do well held in your arms as you feed her with formula from a bottle.

Crying

Crying is the only way babies have to show you what they need and they need you to respond when they cry. Babies cannot cry to manipulate you because they can't yet hold such complex ideas in their minds (see also **Thinking and learning**). Often, at first, parents find it hard to work out what their baby needs. It may help to think about how long it was since the last feed, sleep and nappy change. Has anything happened that might have upset your baby? Is it worth trying a top-up feed? But, especially in the first two or three months, babies sometimes cry for some internal reason that they don't understand and you can't work out. This can be distressing for parents but it helps to know that all babies cry in the early months as their bodies adjust to the world. If they cry a lot, more than three hours a day, it is sometimes called colic. Colic just means unexplained crying. If your baby's cry is unusual or you are worried it is worth having a check-up with your health professional. If there is nothing physically wrong you can remind yourself that it is normal, and that even if the baby doesn't stop crying she knows you are there holding and comforting her. If your baby cries a lot you need to accept offers of help and let your housework go for a while. Your baby will grow out of it and you will learn the best ways to comfort her in time. It is not likely to last more than three months; if it does it is wise to have another health check.

Sometimes a parent becomes really upset by a baby crying. If this happens, going outside with the baby in the pram and going for a walk may help both parent and baby. If this does not help, you need to get help to care for your baby if you can, and take a break until you feel in control of your feelings. Make sure your baby is safe, then go outside in the fresh air, have a cup of tea, ring a friend – whatever helps you to cope – before going back to comfort your baby.

How parents can help

The main thing is to learn what helps your baby. Each baby is different. However some babies are helped by:

- being carried in a baby sling
- sucking a dummy – it is best not to use a dummy until breastfeeding is going well
- music or recordings of noise such as the hum of a washing machine (you can buy these CDs in music and baby shops and online)
- driving in the car
- being pushed in a pram over a slightly bumpy surface (too bumpy and their heads bob all over the place)
- sitting and rocking and singing may help calm both your baby and you.

Spoiling

People often ask about spoiling babies. The answer is simple – you can't spoil a baby with love and care. Babies need you to respond to their cries and to give them warm and loving care. Babies can't wait. They don't know anything about the world or anyone in it. They don't even know that there is anyone there to meet their needs (see 'Object permanence' on p. 13). It is very distressing for them to cry and not to have anyone respond. When you respond promptly they gradually learn that there is someone there to help them and to keep them safe, warm, fed and loved. As they learn this over time they gradually grow in confidence and independence.

A mother's story

When Ellie was around 6 months and not yet holding out her arms to be picked up but smiling and starting to reach for me, I wanted to see if she was ready for a new kind of connection with me. So I put her down on her back and held my hands out over her belly for her to put her hands in mine. I wasn't sure if she would understand yet what I wanted, or if she could physically do it even if she understood. The first time I tried she looked at me intently and after a little while started to flap her arms at her sides. She seemed to be concentrating really hard (not looking at my hands but in my eyes). I waited with my hands out and soon she started to flap her arms around my hands and eventually she managed to get one hand in mine. I held it gently while she worked on the other one and shortly after she got that one in my other hand. She did know what I wanted and she tried really hard until she did it. I gave her big kisses and cuddles. After that first time she got better at putting her hands in mine really quickly.

When babies are learning something new, we take time and wait and watch for their response and give lots of praise for achievement. This is building respectful relationships with your baby as well as new skills.

Growing and learning times

Babies don't grow and learn smoothly; they may have a spurt but then they seem to be marking time. You can see this with their physical growth: they seem to be going along nicely and then suddenly they have learned something new and everything changes. It is the same with mental development. Your baby seems to be going along well and then there will be a week where she is not sick but she seems to regress or go backwards. She may be really unsettled, grizzly, not doing as well as she was and you wonder what you are doing wrong! Then at the end of this time she has suddenly learnt something new. These growing and learning weeks happen around 5 weeks, 8 weeks, 12 weeks, 17 weeks, 26 weeks, 36 weeks, 44 weeks and 53 weeks. Some people call these 'wonder weeks' because babies are learning a wonderful new skill. There is a book about wonder weeks[14] included in References at the end of this book if you want to learn more about these exciting developmental times.

Taking care of yourself

Parenting a new baby is very tiring. It is important for the sake of the baby as well as yourself to take care of your own health – how you feel really affects your baby. This means sometimes letting go of commitments and housework that you would normally do, accepting offers of help and making time to rest when the baby does. New mothers often have some days when they feel a bit 'flat' and weepy. If this continues it can be a sign of postnatal depression. If you are feeling so flat that you can't take an interest in things that you normally enjoy, if you are not sleeping or waking early, losing interest in eating and/or feeling really bad about yourself, you need to seek help from your doctor. Postnatal depression can be treated and babies do best when their mothers are well. While you are getting well, having a partner or good friend to support you and nurture your baby with you will ensure that you both get the support you need.

Family breakup

Family breakup, divorce or separation is difficult for everyone. Everyone grieves. It is most difficult for the child who has no say in what is happening. It can have negative consequences for children, especially the very young.[15] Conflict and stress, and especially separation from their main carer, affects them long before they can understand what it is about. They are at risk of doing worse at school, dropping out of school early and having depression or behaviour problems. There are higher risks if there is antagonism between the parents after divorce, if one parent speaks negatively to their children about the other parent, and if there are financial problems. Older children can make meaning of what is happening and there are fewer risks although family breakup can still have negative effects. However, the good news is that if parents are supportive most children do not have these problems.

Some things that parents can do to help young children cope with family breakup:

- Keep your child's life and routines the same as before, as much as you can.
- Help your child keep in touch with both parents if the relationship is positive; good relationships with both parents are supportive for children.
- For the very young, especially for children under 3, avoid overnight separations from the main carer. Follow your child's cues as to where they feel comfortable.
- Support your child's relationship with the other parent; don't try to get your child to take sides.
- Don't argue in front of your child. Make other times to discuss difficult topics.
- Your child will be distressed and angry sometimes and needs your listening, comfort and understanding. Allow her to express her feelings. Your child may regress to younger behaviour for a while and need more nurturing.
- Children need to know that you will never be separated from parenting and caring for them. If they are older make sure they know the breakup is not their fault.
- Put your child's needs above your own hurt or angry feelings. Get support from an adult friend. Grandparents or another relative may be able to help support your child.
- Talk with a counsellor if your child has ongoing problems or you are unable to work things out with their other parent.

Note: This has been put in the Birth to One section because it is the very young whose needs are likely to be overlooked when parents are stressed, and who are the most vulnerable. For further information about helping very young children after separation see the Guidelines at <http://www.aaimhi.org/viewStory/Policies+and+Submissions>. For older children see Parenting and Child Health at <www.cyh.com>.

Fathers

Fathers can do all the caring things that mothers do for babies except breastfeeding. It brings you closer to your baby if you share in bathing, nappy changing, comforting and all the other caring tasks. Some babies especially like to be gently held and comforted by their fathers. It also brings you and your partner closer together as you both share in the loving care of your baby.

Fathers can be gentle and this is what young babies need. Jiggling or being thrown in the air, for example, may be enjoyed by older children but babies are still adjusting to the world and these activities can be unsettling and even scary for them. Your baby needs to feel safe with you, not scared. As she gets older there will be lots of time for boisterous play.

Note: Jiggling or shaking a baby who is crying is dangerous, even if it stops the crying, as it shakes the baby's brain. Soothing holding and perhaps gentle patting reassures your baby.

One thing that many fathers and babies enjoy is baby massage. Touch is very important to your baby's emotional development and brain development. Baby massage classes can show you how to make the most of your baby's need for touch and are a good way to develop closeness with her. Watch for her cues and stop when she is tired and wants a rest or a change.

If you are the main breadwinner at this time, you can make a great contribution to your baby's wellbeing by supporting your partner in breastfeeding and making sure that she has the space and rest to be able to continue to breastfeed during the first year.

One new mother said: 'The best advice I have heard for new fathers is to take their cue from mothers – not to try to take over but to ask the mother what will help them best in caring for the newborn. This is not to say fathers don't have an important role, but it is very stressful for a mother with so many crazy hormones and new responsibilities not to be in control of where the baby is and how it is being cared for, and supporting her in these early days is likely to work out best for everyone.'

Overview – Birth to One

The list below gives a general idea about what to expect. However, all babies are different and have different life experiences which mean they do things in their own way and time. If you have any concerns about your baby's development, talk with a health professional. You will get reassurance that your baby is doing well or, if there is any problem, your baby will get the help she needs.

Birth to 3 months

- responds to sounds from birth
- watches parent's face when held or feeding, loves eye contact
- grasps a finger when it is put in her hand
- smiles – 5 to 7 weeks
- hands usually open – about 8 weeks
- makes small vocal sounds – starting at 7 to 8 weeks
- starts to follow a moving object with eyes – 8 weeks
- chuckles and squeals with enjoyment – 3 months
- recognises main carer(s) – by 3 months
- starting to take turns making sounds with parent – 3 months
- hands together when lying on back – by 3 months
- can hold a rattle briefly by 3 months

6 months

- responds to image in a mirror
- copies actions such as poking out tongue
- laughs
- rolls over both ways
- shakes a rattle and passes it between hands
- holds out arms to be picked up
- raises head and helps when being pulled to sitting

- makes sounds such as 'da-da'
- pushes self up on arms when on tummy.

9 months

- looks for dropped toy or person who goes out of sight (6–7 months)
- enjoys peek-a-boo games
- responds to words such as own name and 'no'
- copies sounds
- grabs food while being fed
- likely to be crawling, or at least moving around the floor
- sits without support (from 7 months)
- picks up small things between thumb and finger
- passes things from one hand to the other
- waves goodbye, claps hands
- blows raspberries.

12 months

- pulls up to standing, walks holding on to furniture, may be walking
- picks up very small things
- likes to feed self with finger foods, holds spoon
- understands requests such as 'give it to me'
- clear attachment to main carer
- makes good eye contact
- starts to point with index finger
- may say a few words
- gives cuddles
- cooperates when being dressed.

Toys for babies

> **Note:** Toys for babies should not have small parts that can be swallowed – watch out especially for small batteries.

- rattles and things they can make a noise with
- pots, pans and spoons from the kitchen to bang
- books with clear pictures of things they know or animals that you can make the noises for
- plastic rings on a stand
- a sturdy block cart with a strong handle that they can push when beginning to walk
- large cardboard boxes to crawl in and through
- a large ball
- parents are the best playmates for babies – singing, dancing, taking for walks, showing books.

Chapter 2

One to Two

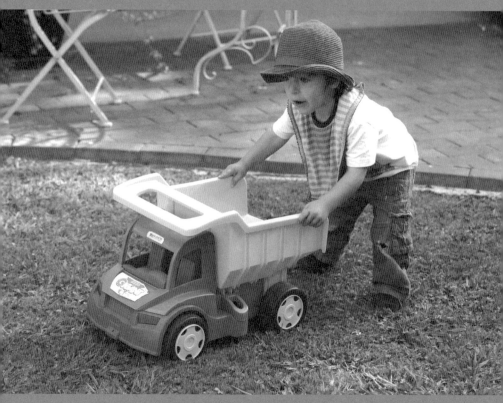

On the move

The major change in the second year of your baby's life is that you see your baby becoming a real individual with his own personality, likes and dislikes and ways of doing things. From the early part of this year he is likely to be up on his feet and going, able to assert what he wants by doing. For most parents this is a really enjoyable time as you see your baby's personality emerging.

When you have a beginning toddler you have a person with a will of his own. There are new challenges of how to respond when your toddler starts to assert his own wishes at one moment, and then wants to be a baby and be comforted the next. He needs to grow and explore but he also needs to feel safe, and he moves backwards and forwards between these needs.

You also have to think about his safety, now that he can be into everything. Check that electrical plugs are covered, that there is no uncovered water in the garden or laundry that he could get into, and that there are no medications within reach, such as in a bedside table or in an open handbag. You have a little person learning to be an individual but he has a lot more to learn about the world before he can manage all the situations he gets into.

Whatever he does, his parents are the most important people in his world and what he wants more than anything else, even if he doesn't always show it, is to please you. Many people think that the year from 1 to 2 is the hardest year of parenting, at least physically. You have to have eyes in the back of your head and be on the go all the time as you encourage your toddler's development and at the same time protect him and everyone else from the consequences of what he doesn't know yet!

Physical development

If your 1-year-old is not yet walking he will probably do so in the next couple of months. Walking takes good balance and at first children walk with their legs wide apart to steady themselves. The next steps are learning to stop when they want to and turn in another direction. Beginning walkers enjoy a toy they can push along. Initially, they do better with a fairly steady toy that won't run away from them. Once they feel steadier on their feet they enjoy carrying toys around, such as their teddies, and having toys that they can pull along as they walk.

Your 1-year-old can crawl up stairs. You can show him how to crawl down stairs and get off a bed safely by turning around and going down backwards (always keeping a watch to make sure he is safe). By about 18 months he can walk up stairs holding on to the rail, putting both feet on each step, with your supervision.

Your child will like to try throwing a big soft ball or rolling it across the floor although he won't be able to catch it yet. He will start to turn the pages in a book, put things down where he wants them to go and build a tower of two blocks. By 18 months he is likely to be walking well and able to squat down to pick up a toy and have a go at kicking a big ball. By 2 years, he is a steady walker who can pick things up without losing balance and is able to walk backwards and to run as well as walk. He might be interested in building a bigger tower with blocks or arranging them into a train. You can probably teach him to suck through a straw and blow out candles.

One-year-olds don't need complicated or expensive resources for their growing and learning. Everything is a wonder to them – keeping their balance while walking or running up and down a slope, following a bird, finding a snail in the garden, playing peek-a-boo around a monument, helping around the house or walking on a plank on the ground. Making plenty of time and space for energetic play every day not only builds their physical and thinking skills but helps to ensure a good night's sleep.

Social and emotional development

One-year-olds have huge learning in social and emotional development. Attachment and separation anxiety (see **Chapter 1: Birth to One**) still loom large in their lives. A 1-year-old is also learning about being a separate individual. For the present he still can't separate out his feelings from yours. If he is cross with you he is likely to believe that you are cross with him and that can be scary for a 1-year-old.

One-year-olds do not usually play actively with other children of the same age. They often like to play near each other and watch others play. When they are playing near others of their own age they need adult supervision because they haven't yet learned about boundaries, and they are likely to try and take what they want in any way they can. You can help them to start learning to wait, take turns and ask, but it will be a couple more years before they can do it well. They often enjoy playing with an older child. They may enjoy going to playgroup with a parent, where there are different things to do and other children around. They need parents to take part in the playing and to watch that children don't hurt each other.

One-year-olds love best of all to play with parents.

Your 1-year-old will enjoy you playing hide-and-seek with him or just hiding behind the curtain and popping out to surprise him. He can learn to trust you best if you support his small forays into exploration and enjoy his success and at the same time accept his need to come back for comfort and reassurance. It is this pattern of coming and going, a little further each time as he feels more secure, that helps your 1-year-old to gradually become confident about going out into the big world as he grows older. He is likely to still need reassurance that you are there at bedtime or if he wakes during the night.

Children learn how to manage their own feelings with your help. To develop confidence and resilience they need you to:

- be reliable and respond to their needs – e.g. reassure and support them when they are afraid
- name their feelings for them – knowing the names of feelings helps to manage them
- talk about feelings as you do your daily tasks – this is a really good investment because it helps your child to be able to recognise feelings and feel comfortable talking about them as they get older e.g. 'I felt really disappointed when I went to buy that book and the shop was shut'
- help them to find ways to cope with frustration e.g. 'shall we try to build up the tower again?'
- help them to learn gradually to wait for some things they want e.g. 'it is Charlie's turn on the swing now, would you like to have a slide first?'
- be there with them as they are trying to manage all these feelings that can overwhelm them.

Some feelings you might want to start naming for your toddler: happy, sad, scared, cross, disappointed, excited, frustrated, upset and so on.

At 14 months Sam was taken to a Wiggles concert – Sam was lucky to be in the front row. But it was too close. When the show started Sam was shaking with fear even sitting on his mother's lap. She took him to the back row so he could watch the show from a 'safe' distance. He loved it. After a while he said he wanted to go a bit closer so they walked slowly down the aisle. Sam decided how far and how fast to go. Gradually he made his way all the way back to the front row for the last few songs and he loved it, dancing along.

Children learn to overcome fears by being able to take things at their own pace and having some control over what happens.

When you have to leave your 1-year-old, even for a short time, let him know that you are going. A good-bye ritual such as waving and saying something like 'see you soon' helps. Parents need to respond to their child's feelings but also reassure him that you know he will be OK; try to show your toddler this by your own confidence. If you look worried, he is likely to think there must be something to worry about! Even if he cries at the time, saying goodbye helps him learn to trust you. It also helps, of course, if you leave him with someone he knows well and feels safe with.

Child care

If both parents are working you will need to look for alternative care for your young child. Grandparents can be a great option for caring for the very young; however many grandparents are working and young parents may live a long way from family supports.

Family day care offers nurture and care in a small group setting in a home-based environment.

Centre-based child care offers different learning opportunities in a larger setting with more children and group experiences. However group child care can be stressful for under threes because of the need to be with groups of children for long periods, before they have learnt many of the skills of playing together.[16] Research has shown that where staff are warm and sensitive and there are enough staff to provide frequent positive interactions with young children, the children are more likely to feel secure and confident and make the most of their learning opportunities.[17]

Visit the child care service you are considering to get an idea of what the experience is like for the children. Some things to look for that will help your child get the most out of the child care experience include:

- a child care setting where they have a special main carer for each child (primary caregiver)
- warm and nurturing staff
- your toddler has plenty of time to bond with the carer before you leave him
- places where children can be on their own as well as places for playing with others
- a small number of children for each staff member, preferably no more than three or four for toddlers
- not too many children in the group
- staff are interested in knowing about your family and incorporating where possible your parenting style (e.g. what your child likes to eat, how you manage meal times and sleep)
- you are welcome at the service any time
- qualified staff.

A few practice sessions at the centre for you and your child are important if you can manage it, followed by leaving your child for short periods at first. It is likely that you will be starting your child in child care at the same time as you go back to work so you may be tired. In addition, young children who have just started child care may find it difficult to settle at night and may want more nurturing from parents to make up for missing them during the day. Try to reduce as many home stresses as you can while you and your child adjust to the new situation. For example, you could decide that you will have a rest yourself while settling your toddler to sleep.

If your child still does not settle after a few weeks, talk with the staff about what other options might exist.

Speech and language

If your child has not started saying meaningful words before he is 1, the words are likely to come in the next couple of months. Once children start speaking, new words come quickly. They also point to things they want, or want to show you. They understand much more than they can say and 1-year-olds can follow simple directions such as 'give it to me' or 'put it on the chair'.

Your 1-year-old can understand 'no'; however he may not have the willpower yet to obey you, even when he knows what it means. You may see a 1-year-old heading towards an electrical power point that he has been told not to touch. He says to himself 'no, no, no' but still heads for the point regardless. It is not disobedience but a stage in learning self-control. He knows what he must do but he can't do it yet. This is one of the reasons why 1-year-olds need constant supervision.

By 18 months most children have a few words and by 2 they know well over 100 words, so parents stop counting! By the time he is 2, your toddler is starting to put words together to make simple sentences such as 'Daddy gone'; 'come here'; 'more milk'. He uses words to ask for things he wants. There is much talking to himself using syllables strung together which are meaningless to adults but is part of the development of language.

Being a beginning talker is very frustrating for toddlers because often they cannot get adults to understand what they are saying. It becomes a guessing game as you try to work out what they mean and is very satisfying for the child when you get it right. Some parents teach their children hand signs for common words to help them let you know what they want before they can tell you in words. You can start this from the time they learn to use their hands to communicate, for example 'Wave bye-bye'. (There is a book about teaching your child sign language by Acredolo et al. under 'Babies' at the back of this book.)

One-year-olds enjoy simple picture books (with and without rhymes), songs and nursery rhymes. These add to their development of language and help prepare them for reading later on and it is important to include some every day. They may like to turn the pages for you and look for things in the pictures. A bedtime story and song is a great habit to start and becomes a special time of unwinding before sleep as well.

Take the time to stop and listen when your toddler is talking to you. Get down to his level and show that you are really interested. When you talk to him, give him time to have a go at answering. Try to repeat what he says and you will soon know if you get it right. When he makes a mistake with a word you can help by repeating it correctly without actually correcting him. For example, if he picks up his ball and says 'boo-boo' you can say 'yes, that is your ball'.

Continue to talk to him about what you are doing as you go about your daily tasks, and naming things that he sees or points to.

Thinking and learning

One-year-olds see the world from their own point of view and think that other people also see it from their point of view. Sometimes this is called egocentric but not in the same negative sense that it is often used by adults. It just means the child's viewpoint of the world comes from what he knows.

They have not yet learned that all their body parts belong to them, so a toddler might stand on a piece of rope and try to pull it without realising that it is his own feet which are holding it. They are often afraid of getting cuts and bleeding, because they think they could lose parts of their bodies. They want a sticking plaster over the cut quickly.

One-year-olds also have not learned that their minds are separate from yours; for example, if they know where they are they think that you do as well. So a toddler who wanders away in a shop does not realise that you don't know where he is.

They don't understand things like time (when things might happen), space (what will fit into what), or size.

They are busy trying and learning all these things. They climb in and out of boxes, over and under obstacles; they push things together and pull them apart; they may try simple puzzles with single pieces and work out which way to turn the pieces to make them fit. They need opportunities to practise, such as utensils to pour with in the bath or sand tray so they are practising what goes into what. You also help when you talk about what they are doing and use words such as under, over, behind, in front of and alongside. Play games with your toddler, pointing to different body parts on you and on him. Ask him to look for things such as 'where is your ball?' Giving toddlers opportunities to do things for themselves is one of the best activities – to push the stroller instead of riding in it, to open the door for you, to carry some of your parcels, and to start taking off their own clothes at bath time.

Your toddler is interested in making things happen, such as using switches to turn things such as lights and the TV on and off. By the end of the year he will probably be copying some things you do, for example, pretending to talk on the telephone.

Toddler Scarlett noticed that when anyone switched the light on, the click of the switch made the Christmas ornament hanging near the switch play a little song. Under the watchful eye of her mother she dragged a chair to the light switch, climbed up and switched the light on and off, experimenting with making the music happen.

One-year-olds delight in learning that they can make things happen, developing a sense of agency.

Play

One-year-olds are getting mobile on their feet and love to push, pull and carry things. Their attention span is usually short so putting some toys away for a while and getting them out again later gives a new interest. They love to explore about your house, what is in cupboards and on shelves, and what can be pulled out or climbed over. They explore through touch so it is a good idea to put your special things out of the way.

Toddlers need lots of opportunities to walk and run and try out their physical skills in safe surroundings. Parks and playgrounds as well as your own backyard are good places to play. Give them opportunities to climb little hills, crawl through and into boxes, climb up and down steps, push and pull toys on wheels and put different things in and out of boxes. They enjoy playing with large balls, pushing and rolling and kicking once they are able to balance well enough.

One toy that most 1-year-olds really enjoy is a simple ride-on toy that they can kick along with their feet. It helps if the first one is easy to get on and off, so those without a high back work well. Follow their lead about what they like to do best. Once they have mastered one skill they want to move onto a new one.

Beginning from the age of 1, swings are popular with children of all ages. They help develop balance and they are comforting.

Sleeping

Some toddlers sleep through the night and some do not. Sometimes it is because life is so exciting that they can't relax at bedtime and want to keep going. Gentle bedtime routines such as a bath, a song, a prayer and a story can help them to relax. Other children are bothered by the separation from their parents and need to know you are still near. It sometimes helps if you use this time to have a rest near your child as he goes to sleep. If toddlers wake in the night and need comfort it might be easier to put a day bed in their room so you can lie down near them and sleep there for a while. Or you could let your child get into your bed if everyone is happy about it. It does not last forever. The main thing is that everyone gets some sleep and that your child is not upset or frightened. (It is not safe for adults to sleep with very young children if they smoke, have been drinking, are very obese or are on any drugs that make them very sleepy — see the SIDS website for more information <www.sidsandkids.org>.)

Eating

Babies are usually good eaters but toddlers tend to become more fussy about food. It is never helpful to force children to eat what they don't want and it can cause ongoing eating problems. Keep offering different healthy foods for your toddler to choose from and don't despair if he wants the same food over and over. This is common in toddlers and they grow out of it. Make sure that there is always something that you know he likes as part of each meal. It also helps if you don't keep a lot of sweet foods in the house that he knows about and it helps even more if you don't eat them in front of him.

If you list what he eats over a couple of days you might be surprised to see that he is getting a reasonable variety, but if you are concerned talk it over with a health professional. Parenting SA <www.parenting.sa.gov.au> has a 'Parent Easy Guide' with more information about feeding toddlers.

One-year-olds are starting to use a spoon for themselves and to hold their own cup to drink without spilling.

Sexual development

From birth, infants get pleasure from their bodies. One-year-olds who have already discovered their hands and feet may discover and explore their genitals. They may touch their genitals for comfort or because it feels good. Young boys may hold onto their penis because they have seen a baby girl without one and are afraid it could come off. Most likely it is simply exploring a different part of their body and it is best if you treat it as natural. You can show this by your attitude and words as you change his nappy. This helps prevent feelings of discomfort about sex which many people from older generations have grown up with. Your 1-year-old may also try to explore his poo when his nappy is off and smear it over available surfaces if you are not watching. He needs to know that poo isn't something to play with but that it is good and shows his body is working well.

Some other things to know about 1- to 2-year-olds

Behaviour

One-year-olds are into everything, try everything, and touch whatever they can with only beginning understanding of what they should and should not do. Because of their need to explore and experiment, you will do best by putting precious things out of reach, rather than continually saying 'no', while also making sure that there are interesting things to do. One-year-olds have a short attention span so you need to be watching for when they get tired of something and into mischief!

They like to learn to help themselves so, as often as you can, leave more time for dressing, bathing and getting ready for going out to allow for enthusiastic helpers. Parenting a 1–year-old is very 'hands-on' as they need you to show and help them as well as tell them what to do. Their day can be full of 'no-es' so it is worth keeping a bit of a count occasionally and seeing how many you can turn into 'yes-es' – telling them what they may do instead of what they may not. For example, you might say 'here is some paper you can draw on' as well as 'we don't draw on walls'.

Your toddler needs to know that you are able to keep him safe from his own behaviour and other dangers. He needs to learn that you will set limits to unsafe behaviour and you will not either leave him or retaliate when he misbehaves. This is how he begins to learn to regulate his own behaviour. First you do it for him (e.g. remove him from a difficult situation); then you do it with him (e.g. help him to clean up a mess); then, over the early years, he learns to manage his own behaviour much of the time. And all the time you talk with him about how he is feeling and what you are doing.

Toddlers learn in the context of their relationship with you. When your toddler has a problem, he needs you to stay with him to help work it out rather than separate from him. He is too young to benefit from methods where he is separated from you, such as putting him on his own in a 'thinking chair' or time out. You may have to take your toddler away from the problem/other children for a time but keep him with you until you can help him to re-direct what he wants to do.

Toilet training

Parents of 1–year-olds often start to think about toilet training. Learning to use the toilet is quite a complex task and most children of this age are not ready to manage it. They have to first be aware of when they need to go, and then be able to know what to do (e.g. get pants down and go to the toilet or potty they are going to use). It is usually easiest if you wait for your child to signal that he knows he has done a wee or poo by telling you, and then encourage him to tell you before it comes. If this happens in the last part of the second year you could try introducing him to the potty. This often works better than the adult toilet which can be scary. Don't make him sit for a long time, but give him encouragement for each part of the process: getting his pants down, sitting and so on. It is important not to let it become a battle or upsetting for your toddler because if toddlers become frightened and hold on to their poo it can hurt when they do pass it and cause an ongoing problem. If your child is not willing, leave it for a while. Most 1-year-olds don't really achieve toilet training although some parents become very adept at noticing when their child needs to do a bowel movement.

Toddlers and activities

When your baby starts to move around you are likely to have lots of ideas about activities for him to join. Activities like playgroup usually work well because they are about children playing as they want to, with close supervision and support from parents.

However, some other activities can be stressful for babies and toddlers and you need to watch your own baby's reaction. If he is being pressured to do something he doesn't like or is afraid of it is better to wait until he is ready for this sort of activity. He will not be disadvantaged by waiting and is likely to be more confident and enjoy it more.

One young mother took her 1-year-old to swimming classes. Her toddler did not like what he was asked to do in the lesson and wanted to stop. He liked the water, however, so she decided to keep going to the lessons, but she just played with him in the water near the other children and he did not do anything he did not like. Swimming 'lessons' became an outing that he really enjoyed.

Forcing young children to do something they are afraid of is likely to make them more fearful.

Fathers

One-year-olds love doing things with dads. They enjoy more boisterous play – but remember to watch for the child's signals that he has had enough; you are much bigger than he is. Also you need to make safe play rules – don't let your 1-year-old hit you or hurt you or damage things in your home. He needs to learn the rules that will help him in play with others later on.

Boisterous play times don't work very well in the couple of hours before bedtime as children get so excited that it is hard for them to relax and go to sleep.

One-year-olds still prefer to go to their main carer for comfort when they are upset and, if this is the mother, sometimes fathers feel hurt that they are not chosen. This is part of the attachment discussed in Chapter 1 and it is the baby and young child's way of feeling safe rather than choosing one parent over the other. Given another year or two you will find that the child will probably just as often choose their father and love the comfort provided.

Overview – One to Two

In this year your baby's individuality develops every day. He is moving into the world as he can now get around well on his own and is starting to be able to use language to express himself. He still has much to learn and while he goes headlong into new experiences he needs you to be ever-watchful to keep him safe. Being a 1-year-old can be dangerous because children try so many things and you need to keep one step ahead of them. It is a good time to give your house a safety check, especially for uncovered water, unlocked medicines and reachable poisons (e.g. under the sink). Driveway safety is also important, particularly when you are backing your car out. Most of all, your toddler needs you to support and enjoy his exploration and to let him come back and be a baby when he needs to.

The list below is a general one to give you an idea about what you might expect in this year. However all children are different and have different life experiences which means they do things in different ways and at different times. If you have any concerns about your toddler's development talk with a health professional. You will either get reassurance that your child is doing well or, if there is any problem, get your toddler the help he needs.

Physical development
▶ begins walking, feet wide apart for balance; later walks backwards and walks carrying a toy
▶ climbs on chairs and up stairs
▶ walks up stairs
▶ runs and jumps

- rides on ride-on toys
- pushes and pulls toys
- holds on and lets go – throws.

Social/emotional development

- is very affectionate and loves cuddles, blows kisses
- still very attached to main carer/separation anxiety
- loves to play near other young children
- not ready to take turns and share without help
- starting to show independence – says 'no'
- needs lots of support from parents.

Speech and language

- starts this year with a few words
- finishes this year with many words and puts words into short sentences
- talks a lot in his own jargon at first
- understands much more than he can say
- enjoys stories and simple rhymes
- turns pages and points to pictures in books.

Thinking and learning

- does simple puzzles
- points to show what he wants
- understands directions e.g. 'put the book on the table'
- starts to learn what groups things belong to e.g. birds, animals, toys
- explores how things work.

Behaviour

- ▶ active play
- ▶ does not yet control impulses (i.e. what he wants to do), needs constant supervision
- ▶ likes to play with cause and effect – switches on toys and TV
- ▶ copies parents
- ▶ likes to help
- ▶ obeys simple requests.

Toys for 1-year-olds

Note: Watch toys for small parts or batteries that could be swallowed.

- ▶ a child-size chair or sofa
- ▶ big ball, to start learning to kick and throw
- ▶ sandpit or sand tray with buckets, funnels, spades and pouring and sifting toys
- ▶ small paddle pool, always used under supervision and covered or emptied when not in use
- ▶ big teddy or doll to carry or push in a toy stroller
- ▶ ride-on toy
- ▶ large blocks
- ▶ simple puzzles
- ▶ posting box
- ▶ push- and pull-along toys

- ▶ nesting boxes for stacking and sorting
- ▶ toy phones
- ▶ CD of nursery songs
- ▶ musical toys such as drums
- ▶ books
- ▶ swing
- ▶ mud and walking in puddles
- ▶ backyards, parks and playgrounds to explore.

Note: Some experts recommend that children under 2 should not see any DVDs. However, there are some DVDs that are specially made for young children that they enjoy and, perhaps, learn from. If you decide to get any DVDs for your young child you need to be sure they are suitable for his age. Watch the DVD with him so you can interpret and reassure as needed. Too much time sitting and watching is clearly not good for young children, who don't have an understanding of what is fact and what is fantasy and who need to explore the world hands-on!

Chapter 3

Two to Three

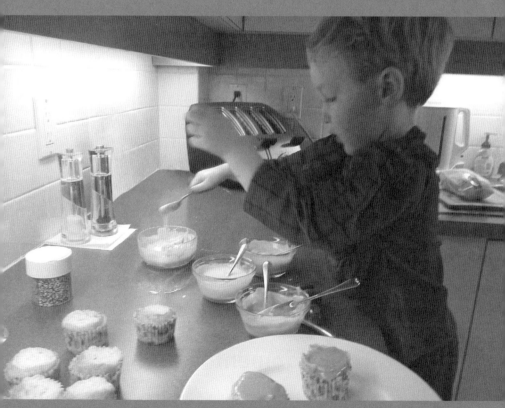

Growing and learning

Even if your child is 2 before you read this book, it is a good idea to read Chapter 2 first. Much of what is in the chapter on 1-year-olds also applies to 2-year-olds.

Two-year-olds are often talked about as 'terrible twos' which makes you think that this is a difficult year for parents. Much of this is due to unrealistic expectations of what 2-year olds are like and what they can do. Two-year-olds, in a way like 14-year-olds, are trying to learn who they are as separate human beings and this can bring some new issues for parents as your previously very agreeable child says 'no' to your suggestions. Sometimes their need to say 'I am a person, I can have a say' even overrides what they really want, so they say 'no' while holding out their hand for the ice-cream. And most parents want their children to be able to be strong enough to say 'no' as they go through life. Now is the time when the foundations for their future individuality are being laid so, rather than being 'terrible', it is an exciting new development. Underneath this, 2-year-olds are still very new to this world and what they need most is their parents' love and approval.

Being different, being oneself, and bringing different skills, talents and interests to a family and community are strengths. Treasure your 2-year-old's exploration and ventures into finding out who she is. What your child brings from her heredity is part of her, but how you respond and guide her is equally important to who she will be.

Physical development

Your child really enjoys her physical skills – running and climbing and exploring. However, she doesn't yet have a sense of what she can do and there will be many falls and bumps. She benefits from some space to run and play such as playgrounds and parks but needs you to be near to ensure that she is safe. Most enjoy speeding along on a ride-on, kick-along toy. Two-year-olds are likely to run away from you, testing their independence, or to jump into a pool because they have no sense of danger, so parents need lots of energy to keep up with them.

Your toddler will soon be able to walk down stairs, as well as up, with both feet to a step, and by the end of the year be able to jump off a low step. She can squat down to play and climb on furniture, especially to get something she wants. She may be learning to walk on tiptoe by the end of the year. She may build a tower of six blocks and turn the pages in a book one at a time. She can grasp a ball if it is rolled to her across the floor; by the end of this year she can catch a big ball as well as throw a ball. Some of her first throws may be over the back of her head so she needs a very adept catcher!

She uses her fingers for smaller tasks and probably uses one hand more than the other. By the end of the year she can copy a circle that you draw as well as copy a line. She will enjoy many more things with her hands such as:

- drawing with a thick crayon
- playing with playdough
- painting with a big brush (painting with water on a fence is a good way to start)
- taking toys apart – watch out for small pieces that she could swallow
- tearing old magazines and gluing pieces on to card or paper
- pouring water and sand with different containers.

Toddlers are likely to spend more time exploring the feel and look of the paint or playdough than drawing or making something. This is the way they learn.

By 3 years, your toddler will be able to take off her clothes and put some of her clothes on, as well as clean her teeth with your help.

Social and emotional development

Two-year-olds are starting to have feelings that they did not have before such as empathy (understanding of others' feelings) as well as jealousy, embarrassment, pride, and guilt and shame when they do something wrong. They need you to help them see that they are not bad people for having negative feelings or for doing wrong things or for making mistakes.

Being 2 is exciting but scary. Being afraid of being away from parents or lost is the toddler's biggest fear. A comforter such as a dummy or blanket that your child is attached to can help with times of separation. If your child has a dummy it is best not to take it away when she is a toddler as it is now that she needs it for comfort as she copes with her expanding world, and when she is separate from you. Most children give it up on their own when they are 3 or 4 and have developed the inner confidence to cope with separations. Dummies are not damaging to teeth until the second teeth come in but it can be helpful to ask your child to take the dummy out when she wants to talk. Some toddlers say they will give up their dummy in exchange for a treat if they are asked. They are not really able to make this decision as they can't think about how they will feel later and it can cause great distress if they are asked to stick to it.

Depending on their experience, toddlers are often afraid of spiders, clowns or masks, dogs and sometimes people who look different. They may also be afraid of being flushed down the toilet.

> Two-year-old Finn says to his mother, 'You have to lift me out of the bath quickly before I go down the drain'.
>
> *Two-year-olds still don't understand about size and what fits into what.*

Toddlers think of themselves in physical terms – 'I am this girl who has long hair, a red dress and a blue bike'. They are not yet able to take turns and share because they haven't fully worked out what is them and what is not them, so it is like taking away a part of themselves to make them share something they think is theirs. This is a good time to have two of the same toy, if you can, and put away anything special when other children come to play. Two-year-olds like to play near other children but mostly play by themselves. Two-year-olds playing together need close adult supervision, as they test how other children react to what they do.

Because they are trying new things without really understanding what they can and can't do, 2-year-olds easily get frustrated and most have tantrums from time or time, or often. Some tantrums are to try to get something they want. In this case you would not want to give in to the request, but the overflow of feelings still needs your support. Sometimes tantrums are 'boilovers', when your child's feelings are really outside of her control. She needs you to show her that you are there to help her through it; that you will neither walk away nor punish her. If your child will not let you hold her, stay near until the tantrum is over and then you can hold her and help her feelings to heal. If you look for when they happen you might be able to prevent some tantrums, for example, not take her to the shop when she is hungry or tired, or divert her when she is frustrated at something she is doing. You cannot prevent them all – they are part of coping with being 2. Telling her the names of feelings is still very important.

Because she is learning independence it works best if you give her many opportunities to make choices and to try things. Simple choices between two things are less confusing than free choice amongst a number of things.

Avoid direct challenges as much as you can. Ask yourself if it really matters or if this is a time when your 2-year-old could be doing it her way. If it does really matter you can often divert a toddler by offering something else or a different activity. Sometimes you need to say 'no' firmly and calmly, move the child away from the problem and wait out the storm if there is one. Giving a simple reason helps: 'No, that is hot'; 'No, we don't hit, it hurts'. Until your 2-year-old can control her own behaviour she needs your active intervention. You don't just tell her: you show her with actions and by showing her that you understand her feelings.

Toddlers want to grow and explore one minute and they want the safety of being a baby the next. Delight in your toddler's independence and exploration, watch over her and welcome her back for reassurance and comfort when she needs it.

Speech and language

Language develops at an amazing rate. You can now understand most of her speech. Your 2-year-old uses her own name to refer to herself, and can name other people she knows well. She can tell you her first and last name, if she has been taught these words. She copies what you say, starts to ask questions and enjoys answering your questions. Examples of her questions may be: 'Who gave me that toy?' 'What said that noise?' If she gets words wrong, instead of correcting her, just follow on with a sentence that says it correctly – she is learning all the time. You could say 'I wonder what made that noise?'

As your child gets closer to the age of 3, she may start saying 'I' when talking about herself. She may be able to talk about how she is different from other people. She can tell you that she is a girl and knows if another child is a boy or a girl, usually by what they are wearing. By about two-and-a-half she can use sentences with several words. Her understanding of words that she knows is good and you can ask her to do something with two suggestions at a time. For example: 'Can you get your milk from the fridge and bring it to me?'

Give simple explanations to help her understand you. If you just say 'no' she may misunderstand. For example, suppose you are gardening and you say 'no' when she pulls up a flower as she tries to help you with weeding. She doesn't know if you mean 'No, don't walk on the garden' or 'No, don't pull up anything' (when she has just seen you pull something up), or 'No, that is my special flower, you can pull up this weed'.

She enjoys stories and songs and these should be part of every day. She can name or point to things she recognises in pictures and likes to say or sing songs and nursery rhymes with you. You can help her language development by reading to her, talking to her, listening to her and responding, and showing her that reading matters as you go about your daily tasks. For example, 'That red sign says stop, so I had better stop'; 'I am just writing a list of things I need to get at the shop'. If you make the alphabet song one of her nursery songs, she will get to know the letters of the alphabet as she sings.

Thinking and learning

Toddlers are starting to learn things that are beginning mathematics such as understanding patterns and groups; for example, they may put all the spoons together. They can help you sort things by colour, such as blocks or pegs, and by shape. If they help set the table they learn that there is one knife and one fork for one person. If you give them water or sand and different containers to pour with, such as plastic jugs and funnels, they can practise what fits into what as they learn about shapes and sizes.

By the end of the year they know what '1' means and may be able to correctly count three things as well as say numbers up to 10 or more.

They know about over and under, fast and slow, loud and soft, big and small. Playing games that include these ideas help children to learn about them in practical ways. You can play games that include running fast and then slowly, put toys in boxes, hide under tables, and listen for loud and soft sounds. Active experience really helps children to expand their knowledge.

Two-year-olds are fascinated by the world they live in – how their shadow changes, how the wind blows bubbles up in the air and the tiny creatures that live in the garden.

There are lots of things that 2-year-olds don't yet know that might surprise you. They cannot separate fact from fantasy, and they don't understand abstract ideas such as time and death. This means that if a pet dies, for example, they do not understand why it is not there tomorrow. And if you say you are going out and will be back in the afternoon it is not meaningful. It helps them to understand if you talk to them in very practical terms, such as 'I will be back after you have your sleep'.

You can help them gradually sort out fact from fantasy by telling them what is not real, what is alive and what is a story. If they think there is a monster in their bedroom, don't go looking for it because that says that you think there is a monster to look for – just tell them that monsters are not real.

> When Anna bumped into a table and hurt her head she said, 'Naughty table!'
>
> *Toddlers believe that things can act as if they are alive.*

They still see the world from their own point of view and think that other people feel and see things the same way they do. So if your 2-year-old says 'I hate you', which she might do if she is very angry, she is likely to think that you hate her too, which is very frightening for a 2-year-old. They still haven't learned that their minds are separate and they think you know what they are thinking.

Children are learning who they are as separate people and developing their own special identity in many ways. You can help them by talking about comparisons. You can talk about differences between people such as different cultures, and different likes and dislikes such as 'I like coffee and Daddy likes tea and you like milk'.

Toddlers explore the world when they are taken for walks around the block, to parks, and near building works and railway lines. Talk about what you see. Let your toddler have time to walk on walls holding your hand, look at ants and snails, or stamp her feet in puddles. Play 'follow the leader' around the house or garden, when she can be leader. Try hiding surprises under a cushion, or move the surprise from one cushion to another and let her find it. Follow her lead about what she likes to do.

Jani who is nearly 3 asks, 'Do you like this one, Mummy. Is this your favourite?'

Two-year-olds are starting to separate themselves from others and see that different people like different things.

Play

Toddlers are starting to learn to explore and to use drawing, painting and modelling materials. They tend to like bright colours best. They love copying your tasks so your broom, vacuum cleaner, rakes and hoes are all good playthings. They also love dressing up and playing make-believe games – both as favourite heroes from stories and as grown-ups from real life (in your old clothing). Op shops can be excellent sources for dress-up clothing.

They still enjoy their ride-on toys and carrying toys around with them, or pulling them in carts. A sandpit can be a source of enduring fun with different toys, kitchen pots and pans, and a hose from time to time. Sandpits need to be covered at night and when not being used to deter visits from cats.

Two-year-olds play near other children but need good supervision because they have not learned the skills of sharing and taking turns and how to consider others.

If they have the opportunity, two-year-olds enjoy playing simple computer games and this helps to familiarise them with computers as well. However active play, outdoors when possible, is still most important for their development and encourages a good night's sleep. They not only get to exercise their muscles; they test their courage and skill as they climb and explore and learn lots about thinking as they work out how high a rock is to jump off, whether they can fit through small openings or how many steps they can climb up. Most of all they like to play with parents. Chasing games, follow the leader and hide-and-seek are popular with two-year-olds.

Sleeping

Bedtime is a separation from parents and from all the things a 2-year-old has enjoyed during the day so many 2-year-olds find it hard to relax and go to sleep. Having a regular bedtime routine is very important (see Chapter 2) and you will probably find that your toddler insists on doing things exactly the same way each time. She might want the same story, the same song and the same glass of water that she has every night. This helps her to deal with the separation and fears of the night, just as adults like having something familiar when dealing with the unknown. She may also need the reassurance of knowing you are there if she wakes in the night.

Eating

Two-year-olds like to keep to their routines and may not take to new foods. Keep offering different healthy foods but accept that she will try them when she is ready. Make sure that foods she does like are always available; don't try to make her eat what you think she should eat, or to go without if she doesn't eat a particular food. As long as your toddler doesn't get a lot of junk food or sweet drinks such as cordials, you will probably find she is getting an adequate diet if you keep a list of what she eats for a couple of days. Battles about food can cause ongoing problems and need to be avoided.

Sexual development

The 2-year-old, like the 1-year-old, is still interested in exploring her body, and running around without wearing clothes when she can. She is also interested in other people's bodies and how boys and girls are different and how people go to the toilet. She will watch her mother and father in the shower with interest. Boys may still be worried about losing their penis when they see girls without one, and need reassurance that boys and girls are different and both have special body parts. Two-year-olds often touch their genitals for comfort when they are worried or stressed. Telling them the names of all their body parts is helpful for later on and often comes more naturally when they are very young.

Some other things to know about 2- to 3-year-olds

Behaviour

Your toddler deals with the bigness of the world by sticking to what she knows. She is likely to resist changes to her routines, toys or food. Having what she knows around her helps her to cope with all the new things entering her life.

Behaviour is the way toddlers communicate how they feel. They are not yet capable of really expressing their needs and feelings in words, so when you respond to behaviour you need to do it on two levels:

- how you react to what they are doing
- how you respond to what the behaviour means.

For example, if your child bites another child it is an opportunity to help her learn that biting is not OK and also for you to hear the message behind the bite. So you might say 'I can see you need help. We don't bite because biting hurts. Were you feeling cross because Max took your toy car? Can you say to Max "No, my car"'. You might then talk about Max's feelings as well. As stated earlier, toddlers playing together need close supervision.

Toddlers need lots of opportunities to choose. Complicated choices confuse them and they do better if you give very simple choices between only two things (e.g. 'Do you want to wear the red top or the green top?')

They are not yet able to put themselves into your shoes and think about what you want, so when they seem to be wanting to be the boss it is really about finding out who they are, not trying to get at you. Your toddler needs to try out being individual so think before you say 'no' to her. Is it necessary or can she follow her own way? There are many, many times when you will have to say 'no' to help her learn to be safe and to get along with others. Where possible try to tell her what she may do, instead of or as well as what she may not – for example 'I know you can talk quietly' instead of 'Don't shout'. It also helps to play fun games about saying 'no': 'Are cows green?' 'No'. 'Does the doggy say, moo?' 'No'. And so on.

Discipline

All children need limits for their behaviour to help them feel and be safe and to get along with other people. In the toddler years parents really start to think about how they discipline their children. Discipline means teaching, not punishment. Sometimes there must be consequences as a result of a child's behaviour so she can learn from it. Children, however, don't need to be hurt emotionally or physically in order to teach them how to behave. For example, if a young child makes a mess she can help you clean it up; if she throws a hard object (because she is learning to throw) you can take it away and give her something soft; if she hurts other children maybe she needs to stay away from them and only be with you for a while until she can manage her feelings.

When responding to your child's behaviour, ask yourself what is the message behind the behaviour?

Below are some examples of toddler behaviour, the message that may be behind it and some suggested options for parents to consider.

Table 3.1. Toddler behaviour

Toddler behaviour	Message	Parent response
Doesn't share a toy with another child	I am doing what is right for my age, and I haven't yet learned about what is me and mine	• Check your expectations for your child's age • Provide similar toys for both children, or assist one to find something different
Tantrum in the evening	I am stressed, tired, unwell, frustrated, bored …	• Is it something I could prevent by better planning? Look at what happened before and after tantrum and plan e.g. earlier meal, comforting activity such as a story
Throws blocks when the tower she is trying to build falls down	I am trying something I can't do yet and I can't manage my feelings	• Talk about her feelings to show you understand • Do it with her until she can manage it • Tell her that blocks are not for throwing
Hits you when you are feeding the baby	I am feeling unloved, bad, guilty, angry, sad	• Talk about the feeling • Try to meet the need • Show other ways to express the feeling e.g. use words (and don't allow her to hit) • Find something to interest her during feeding

Note: Our responses to children's behaviour are always influenced by our own feelings and some things they do really press our own buttons. This is often related to what was done to us as children (or sometimes what sort of a day we have had). It is important to be aware of this (see title by Bonnie Harris listed in 'Early childhood resources' on page 192). Our parents, like us, were doing the best they could with the knowledge they had, but we know lots more now and we need to learn from any mistakes they made, not repeat them.

New baby

One of the biggest stresses in the life of a 2-year-old is likely to be the arrival of a new baby. In time the new baby will be a playmate, friend, support in times of trouble and someone to enjoy life with. But for now the new baby is taking the toddler's place in your time, thoughts – and to her mind – love. Toddlers see love as the amount of time you spend with them and the time that was devoted solely to your toddler now has to be shared. Sometimes she has to take second place because babies' needs are immediate. She needs you to help her to know that she is still as special as she ever was and to understand that she will feel hurt and sad and angry sometimes.

How parents can help
- Make arrangements for your toddler to be cared for by someone she knows well in familiar surroundings during the birth.
- Make some special time each day for your toddler after the baby comes.
- Don't ask your toddler to do something hard around the baby's birth such as move from her cot to a bed or start toilet training.
- Understand if your toddler misbehaves that she is showing you she is unhappy. Let her know that you understand how she feels

but you won't let her push the baby or throw her milk on the floor. If you punish her she thinks that it proves you don't love her as you did before.

- Don't leave a toddler alone with a baby, especially in the bath – accidents happen.
- Read stories about new babies where there are some negative feelings expressed as well as positive ones; this shows her that you understand how she feels.
- Let her help you with the baby.
- Try to work something out for feeding times such as a baby doll for her to feed, a DVD that she can sit near you and watch, or a special toy to play with.
- Sometimes choose the toddler. Make times when Dad or someone else cares for the baby while you do something special with the toddler, for example, go for a walk, go to the shop for a milkshake, or have a story. Be careful about the number of times you ask someone to care for the toddler while you look after the baby.

Note: It is a good idea to not make too much of the baby's coming a long time in advance. Six months can be a long time for a toddler to worry about something that she doesn't really understand.

Toilet training

When your child goes for longer periods without wetting, wakes up dry after a sleep and starts to let you know when she is doing a poo or wee, she may be ready to start toilet training. Try putting her on a potty when she wakes up dry after a sleep and see if she has some success. It is usually better not to use the big toilet at first because she doesn't yet understand that she can't go down the toilet when you flush it. Give her praise for sitting on the potty even if she doesn't do anything and for any of the tasks that she can do such as pulling down her pants. If you turn on a tap with the sound of running water it sometimes helps her to get started. If this goes well you could try putting her into pants during the day rather than nappies as these feel different and will remind her. Then, if she doesn't object, you could remind her to go on the potty when you think she needs to. Many children more or less toilet train themselves when they are ready, but there will be accidents for a while and it is important not to let your child feel bad about this (as she will if you are too disappointed at a slip-up). If she finds it all too difficult or gets upset give toilet training a break for a while.

Children and the media

Some things you should be aware of when watching television are:

- Young children are not able to judge distance, so something on the news happening far away can seem like it could happen to them
- They don't understand what is real and what is not real
- A lot of fast-moving images, as in some cartoons, can be very unsettling.

Watch TV with your child. Limit TV time to programs that are suitable for the very young. Television is absorbing and exciting and children learn lots from watching but it is not active, creative, child-controlled play so set limits on what and when they can watch.

Temperament

Our temperament is our natural way of approaching and reacting to the world. It affects how children manage in different situations. The way parents and carers relate to children's different temperaments is the most important predictor of how well they will do.[18] There is nothing wrong with different temperaments. We are all different and it would be a boring world if we were all the same. We need to help children make the most of their temperaments and to learn how to adapt to different situations.

Children do best if there is a good fit between parenting and their natural temperaments. Sometimes this is easy – for example, if you are a loud, boisterous household and you have a very active, boisterous child, you are likely to enjoy your child's temperament and she will do well. If you are a very quiet, self-contained parent you need to make an effort to understand and support your active, noisy child. Parents need to adjust to their child's temperament needs, as young children cannot adapt to ours.

Some of the temperament types that are most useful to know about are:

* easy
* very active
* distractible
* sensitive
* slow to warm up
* persistent.

Some children might fit best into one of these categories, but most children are a mixture of them all. Below is a guide to start you thinking about what your child's temperament might mean and how you might best support her.

Table 3.2. Temperament style

Temperament style	Child's behaviour	Parent response
Easy	• Sunny natured, not easily upset • Goes along with what parents want most of the time	Parents usually hope for this kind of child. However there is a risk that an easy, non-demanding child gets overlooked and may not get her needs met. This child needs you to be careful to notice and ask what she needs and to make sure her needs are met. Help her to learn to ask for what she needs.
Very active	• Always on the go, likely to get into difficult situations physically, can't sit still very long • May be good at sport and outdoor activities	This child needs room to run and opportunities for energetic activities every day. Don't expect her to sit for long periods doing quiet tasks. You can gradually teach her by giving short, quiet activities and stopping when she needs a break. Gradually make the activities longer, and have lots of breaks in between.
Distractible	• Easily distracted from a task • Likes to try lots of different things without necessarily finishing one • May be flexible, open to new ideas	Most 2-year-olds have short attention spans so it is hard to pick this quality at such a young age. This child needs lots of different things to try and to explore. When there is something that needs more attention, she needs a quiet place without distractions and support to keep at the activity, such as making a game of it, or ideas to keep it interesting.

→

Temperament style	Child's behaviour	Parent response
Sensitive	• Easily upset, fussy, may be distressed by noise or sudden changes • Doesn't take well to change • May be very perceptive and understanding of others as she grows	This child needs you to be aware of her sensitivity, to take changes slowly. Give her time to adjust, be with her and support her as she learns. Adjust your expectations to her pace.
Slow to warm up	• Takes time to change and relate to new people and places • May be a loyal and rewarding friend	Introduce changes slowly. Don't push her into new situations. Avoid labels such as 'shy'. With practice and support she will gradually take on new ideas and relationships.
Persistent	• Finds it difficult to move between activities • Sticks at the same thing and resists changes (obviously a very good quality in many ways, especially for getting things done)	Give warning of changes such as meals or going out. Help her to learn to put an activity aside and come back to it.

Note: Temperament is present from birth. I have discussed it in this chapter on 2- to 3-year-olds because this is the age when parents are thinking about how to help their child with all the demands of the world. However, knowing your own child and what works best for her is important at every age.

Overview – Two to Three

Two is a year of big changes as your baby is becoming a child. She wants and strives for independence one moment and needs to cling for comfort the next – both are equally part of being 2 years old and being human. We can't move forward until we are sure we are secure where we are. Two-year-olds live for the here and now. They see things from the viewpoint of their own wants and wishes. They have lots of words and one of the roles for parents of 2-year-olds is to use those words to help them start to make meaning of what happens in their lives. When children can make some sense of what is happening, life is not so unexpected or daunting, and you are helping your 2-year-old to get there as you explain and predict and give words to happenings and feelings.

There will be many ups and downs in your relationship with your 2-year-old. Whenever you have an issue that causes upset to you or her, the most important part is the getting together and reconnecting afterwards.

Don't forget how important you are. Your 2-year-old sees herself in the mirror of your eyes. If you have faith in her, believe she is capable and she can get where she wants to go, she will believe that too. If you call her a wimp, or naughty or bad she will believe that as well. So let her know all the time that you love her and you have faith in her and you are setting her on the pathway to being whatever she wants to be.

The list below is an overview of some of the new learning that your child will have over this year. However all children develop differently; they gain new skills in their own time, both because of what they have inherited and even more because of the kind of environment and experiences they have. If you are worried about any aspect of your child's development, talk with a health professional. If she needs help in any area, it is best to get it sooner rather than later, as children's brains and bodies have much more scope for learning when they are very young. And if there is no problem it will be good for you to be reassured.

Physical development

▶ runs, climbs and explores

▶ walks down stairs, as well as up, with both feet to a step

▶ jumps off a low step

▶ walks on tip-toe

▶ builds a tower up six blocks

▶ turns the pages in a book one at a time

▶ catches a ball if it is rolled to her across the floor, as well as throws a ball

▶ catches a big ball by 3.

Social/emotional development

▶ wants to be a separate individual and says 'no' to show she is different

▶ still needs lots of comfort from parents

▶ some separation anxiety – may be afraid at night

▶ likes to do things in the same way, often resists changes

▶ plays near but usually not with others of the same age

▶ usually not yet ready to share and take turns

▶ needs to be supervised when playing with others (to avoid children hurting each other).

Speech and language

▶ uses own name to refer to herself

▶ can tell you her first and last name

▶ starts saying 'I' when talking about herself

- can say what sex she is and knows if another child is a boy or a girl
- starts to ask questions and to enjoy answering your questions
- uses sentences with several words
- speaks clearly enough for parents to understand what she is saying
- starts to understand ideas such as fast and slow, loud and soft, big and little.

Thinking and learning

- starts to put things into groups
- can understand what 'one' means and may be able to count three things
- cannot separate fact from fantasy, believes that things such as rocks are alive and can act
- doesn't understand abstract ideas such as time
- thinks that other people feel and see things the same way she does
- hasn't learned that her mind is separate and she thinks you know what she is thinking.

Behaviour

- wants to be independent one minute and a baby the next
- wants to do things her own way
- may have tantrums as can't yet manage strong feelings
- copies parents
- wants to please parents.

Toys for 2-year-olds

> **Note:** Watch toys for small parts or batteries that could be swallowed.

▶ ride on kick–along toys
▶ toys to pour and float in the bath, bath crayons, bubble bath
▶ toys to push and pull
▶ some may be ready for a tricycle
▶ simple toys that come apart and can be put together
▶ lots of wooden blocks
▶ big balls
▶ DVDs for toddlers to watch with parents
▶ CDs with nursery songs
▶ paints, crayons and large paper
▶ sandpit or tray with pouring and digging toys
▶ paddle pool and hose on the lawn on hot days
▶ playdough
▶ jigsaws and posting boxes
▶ dress–ups and household equipment such as brooms, dusters, tools, garden implements
▶ DUPLO® blocks
▶ floaties for the beach or pool (with supervision)
▶ bubble pipes and blowers
▶ swing.

Chapter 4
Three to Four

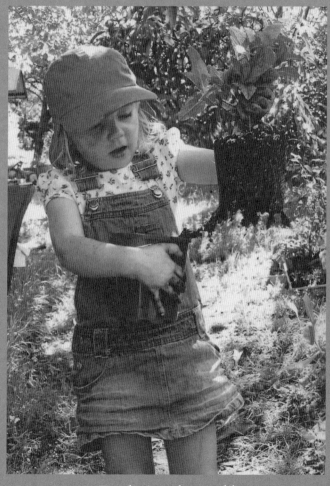

Exploring the world

Three to four may be a more settled time for your child as he can understand much more about his world and use language to help his understanding and express his feelings. He can do more for himself and he is more in control of his actions and his feelings. He is much more capable physically. Best of all, he now has confidence and understanding that he is loved and secure and he will be much happier to venture out on his own, to start to play cooperatively with others. You can enjoy conversations with him and delight in his newfound sense of confidence and his joy in the world. If all is going well for them, 3-year-olds are easy to get along with.

Physical development

Three-year-olds love activity and trying out different climbing and play equipment as well as natural features of parks and playgrounds. They can jump off steps and rocks, walk along walls, walk up stairs with alternate feet and do short hops on one foot. They begin to be able to pedal on a tricycle and balance on a scooter. They can throw a large ball and catch it.

They are mostly able to undress and dress themselves, including managing buttons if the buttons are not too small. They can feed themselves. They are starting to use scissors to cut and they can copy a circle and a vertical and horizontal line if you draw one for them.

Boys in our society are often better at the skills that need strength and whole body movement, while girls may be better at things like drawing and craft activities. However this is largely due to practice. Parents often give girls activities like cutting, pasting and drawing, while boys are likely to have more encouragement to kick and throw balls.

You can help your 3-year-old by giving him time and opportunities to do things for himself. He needs lots of time every day for outdoor play, and space for running, climbing and exploring. Your 3-year-old will like to play on things he feels confident about, as well as experience some challenges. Some children are less adventurous than others and need more encouragement. Doing something well encourages them to try more.

Lots of throwing and catching balls for both girls and boys helps them to develop the skills they need for the future; so do activities that involve hand and finger skills such as drawing, painting and building with blocks.

Social and emotional development

Three-year-olds are more likely to tell you about feelings rather than have a tantrum as they did at 2. They like to please parents and enjoy helping adults. They are very sensitive to what parents think about them and judge themselves by what parents say about them. Encouragement and loving parenting helps children to develop good self-esteem as well as helping their relationships with others. It is important, when a child feels he is in trouble, to reconnect with him so that he is not overburdened with shame or guilt.

Three-year-olds still have fears, often related to stories or images on film or television. They still don't really understand what is real and what is not real. You can help by watching programs with your child and talking about what he sees. Talk with him about the stories you read together, answering any of his questions.

If your 3-year-old has a comfort toy or dummy, he probably needs it much less now and will soon be ready to give it up. He may still want it at times of stress. It works best if you let him give it up in his own time, rather than persuade him. However, you could suggest that he puts the comforter on a shelf where he can get it when he wants it, rather than have it all the time.

As your 3-year-old has more self-confidence to do things on his own and to be apart from you for longer periods, he is also more interested in other children and the beginnings of learning to be a friend which is so important to his future social development. There is more about this in the section on **Play**.

Some 3-year olds, especially only children, have an imaginary friend. This friend is a playmate and may be blamed for any accidents that happen around your child. This friendship naturally disappears as your child gets older and develops real friendships. In the meantime, woe betide you if you sit on the imaginary friend's chair!

Speech and language

Three-year-olds usually know more than 1000 words (many more than you can count) and speak clearly enough for other people as well as their own parents to understand them. However, there are a few sounds that are harder to say and it may take up to a couple of years longer for some children to learn to say *ch, l, r, s, sh, th, v, y,* and *z*. They can tell you what colour things are and what things belong together, such as what are animals, what is food and what are clothes. They can also talk about what things do and what you use things for, and tell you their name, sex and age. They use more complex sentences including prepositions such as in, behind and under. They love to talk and ask questions, so many questions in fact that it can be a bit daunting for parents. You may have to ask for a short rest from time to time, but helping children find answers is great learning for them.

Your 3-year-old is likely to copy what you say. So if you say something like 'I will be really cross if you don't stop doing that NOW' you might expect to hear your 3-year-old say 'Mummy, I will be really cross if you don't get my breakfast NOW!'

Three-year-olds love stories, including funny ones, and simple jokes, poems and rhymes. As you read to them they are getting an idea that the words on the page tell a story and about how books work – all this is part of learning about language and reading.

You can help your 3-year-old by showing him that words are all around him. Talk with him about what you are doing and what he is doing, about the stories you read to him, about what might happen in the stories, about what he did today and what he might do tomorrow. Point out some letters as you read to him if he likes you to, and show him street signs and shop signs. He might be able to find the first letter of his name in signs. He might also help you shop by recognising and picking out your usual groceries in the supermarket. Answer his questions as well as you can; if you don't know the answers look them up or ask someone and let him see you do this. Try making up some stories where he fills in the missing word and encourage him to tell you simple stories.

Thinking and learning

Three to 4-year-olds are making big steps in their thinking. They are learning that the things around them are not magic and can't hurt them. They are learning what is real and what is not real and that their minds are separate. When your 3-year-old makes a mistake and tells you that 'the big bad wolf did it' he now knows that his mind is separate and you can't tell what he is thinking. When he tells you things that are not true he is practising this new learning. You can help him by letting him know the difference between stories and facts, and that both have their place.

Your 3-year-old is starting to do drawings that really mean something. He can draw a simple person, most likely just a head with two stick legs.

By the end of the year your child can count up to five or more. He can sort things by colour, such as buttons or pegs, and can line up things in order of size or put nesting boxes together correctly. When fruit is shared and each child gets one piece he is learning about numbers. When he sees how plates are put on the table and the routine of what happens each day in the morning and at bedtime he is learning about patterns. When he sees that some people in his family like chocolate ice-creams for a treat and some like strawberry, and his father buys the right ones for the right people, he is learning about collecting and using information.

He is learning about using symbols and including them in his play, for example, the broom may be a horse, a spear or a very long magic wand! Using symbols is a very important part of his learning.

His understanding of time is still developing. He can tell you things that he has done but does not have a good understanding of when it was in relation to now, or of how long it is until his birthday, for example. It helps not to give promises too far ahead unless you are happy to have your 3-year-old asking daily 'Is it my birthday yet?'

Talk about colours and numbers and size as you do things: 'Shall we have a brown egg or a white egg?' 'I wonder if the water in the jug will fit into the glass.' 'Do you want a red pencil or a blue pencil?'

Play

Your 3-year-old will probably want to have another child over to play and this is a really helpful way to have children learn the skills of friendship. Having two similar toys such as two tricycles, or an activity that can be done together such as building with blocks, is good for when friends come to play.

Three-year-olds love playing pretend games which involve dressing up, taking on adult roles or roles out of stories and fairy tales.

> Tom, when he's playing with friends, says, 'You be Captain Hook and I'll be Jake – then we have to find the doubloons'.
>
> *Symbolic play is important for children's thinking and learning as well as being enjoyable.*

Your 3-year-old is likely to want to play with others of his own age. Three-year-olds are starting to take turns with toys and wait for their turn without getting upset, although there will be many times when they don't want to share special things.

> Lennie, who is just 3, has started saying to his mother when he gets a new toy, 'The kids will enjoy this'.
>
> *Three-year-olds are starting to learn to predict how others will think and respond to them.*

As they learn more about themselves they are also learning to relate to other children's feelings and to sometimes offer help to another child in trouble. Some of the time they still play near rather than with each other; sometimes they play separately but with the same equipment; and sometimes they can play co-operatively together, sharing toys and building on each other's ideas for the game. Playing together helps children to learn about getting on with each other and sorting out problems. Parents can help children gain play and problem-solving skills by helping each child to talk about their own feelings and then to listen to how the other child feels, so they have more chance of working out a solution that is helpful to both of them. When you play with your child you also help him to develop the skills of playing with others.

> Zach has Lucien over to play. Lucien is playing with some trucks. Zach says 'Lucien, come in the bedroom, come play in the curtains'. Lucien says 'No, I don't want to'. Lucien continues to play with the trucks and Zach does a drawing.
>
> Zach and Vincent are playing in the sand on the beach. Vincent wants to make a sand castle with a moat and Zach offers to help. Zach fills up buckets with water and passes them to Vincent to pour in the moat.
>
> *Sometimes children play together because they both like the same game. Sometimes a child will make an offer to contribute to the other's game – this is one of the skills of friendship they are learning. Sometimes they play separately.*

They love to help you with adult activities such as cooking and gardening. They are also interested in simple crafts, drawing and building with blocks. And of course they love outdoor play and need some outdoor playing time every day. Many children enjoy simple games on the computer and are starting to develop computer skills.

Young children love rough and tumble play with their parents, often with dads. It is up to the parents to set the rules about not hurting anyone, and not destroying the furniture! These are not games for the hour or two before bedtime because 'hyped-up' children don't easily settle into sleep.

Sleeping

Three-year-olds are becoming more confident to sleep without needing support from parents, although they may have nightmares and need comforting. Usually bedtimes and sleep are easier than for younger children as your 3-year-old can hold his good memories of you in his head if he wakes in the night. He knows you are there and will come back. A relaxing bedtime routine is still helpful and he may be able to tell you what will help him sleep better. He may like his door open, or shut, or like a night light or darkness. He might like you to pop in a couple of times after he is in bed. If he does wake in the night and want you, you can put a small mattress and sleeping bag by your bed so he can come and be near you without disturbing your sleep too much.

Eating

Most 3-year-olds are getting more adventurous with food and will usually at least try new things that you suggest, although some children are fussy eaters until they are at school. (In the early school years, when they are going to friends' houses and eating with other children, they are likely to eat food at their friends' houses that they would not eat at home.) It is better not to force the issue or make your child go without eating if he doesn't like what you have chosen. Keep presenting small amounts of new foods but also give him some options that you know he likes.

Sexual development

Three-year-olds are likely to be interested in each other's bodies and may play games that involve looking at each other with their clothes off. This is a part of their play but should not dominate it. They should not have sexual knowledge beyond their years. They may ask you about how babies get out and about differences between boys and girls. A simple, truthful answer giving just the amount of information that children want will help them to start getting a healthy understanding of sexuality before they are exposed to the sniggers that they are likely to meet at school. Having good information gives children confidence. You could say in response to a question about why girls don't have a penis something like: 'Boys and girls are different and they both have special parts. Boys have a penis and girls have a special place called a vagina.' Getting a simple book for children and looking at it with them is a good way to start answering questions and giving your children information.

Children may masturbate because it feels good to them, or for comfort when they are worried or frightened. This is an age when you can tell them that it is not something that people do in public.

If your child is doing it a lot you might think about what worries he has that you could help with.

Children learn their attitudes to sexuality from their parents. If you feel comfortable about the sexual parts of their bodies they are likely to also. They also need to see that you are glad your child is a boy, or a girl, and that you respect both men and women.

Some other things to know about 3- to 4-year-olds

Laughing

Having a sense of humour is important for children, especially when things are tough. We can help them by sharing what we enjoy and the way we can (sometimes) find something to laugh at even when things go wrong.

Adults sometimes laugh at children, perhaps because they enjoy what the child is doing or saying and sometimes because they think the child's natural behaviour or question is funny. By the time they are 3 children can understand about and feel embarrassment and shame. They know when they are being laughed at and it triggers embarrassment and reluctance to take risks that can be lasting. Some children are more sensitive than others, but no-one likes being laughed at. You can explain to children about the different kinds of laughter including laughing together and laughing for happiness, and that these are more likely motivations for laughter than laughing due to ridicule. However, it is also important to get adults to understand that it is as unkind to laugh at children who are trying to learn or do something as it is to laugh at adults and can be very discouraging.

> When her mother's friend asked Janie to sing a song she said, 'No you'll laugh' and the friend said, 'No I won't. I promise I won't laugh'. Janie said, 'No you will laugh and laugh'. Eventually she did sing a song and the friend didn't laugh.
>
> Janie's mother explained that no-one ever laughed at Janie but sometimes she made people so happy by her singing that they smiled so big they ended up laughing. But it was only because they thought she was such a good singer. Janie wasn't convinced.
>
> *Children by the age of 3 are learning to predict how others will react to them and to avoid situations where they feel uncomfortable.*

Behaviour

Three-year-olds are usually friendly and helpful if they are not too tired or unhappy. You can give simple explanations of why you want them to do something, giving them a hand if they need it. You can also expect them to be learning to do things to help themselves – pack up toys, listen to others' points of view and generally be reasonably helpful. However, they are still very young and can get waylaid by all sorts of other interesting things in the middle of doing something for you. Usually, 3-year-olds want to please parents and will respond to your explanations.

Discipline

Discipline is about teaching and 3 is a good age to be teaching children some of the skills they will need to make their way as they start doing more things away from home and spend more time playing with other children. Teaching involves telling them how to do what they need to know, showing them how and coaching them if they get it wrong at first.

From when your child is very young, you will be teaching him to think about how the other person feels. This is good for play and social skills. You might teach your child that if he wants to talk he needs to wait for a space in the conversation before saying 'Excuse me' and putting his request. Teach him to ask when he wants to play with something another child is using. If he gets it wrong often, you can show him and then let him practise.

When a child persistently disobeys, you need to look for a cause. Think about what happened before and what happened after. Can you prevent it happening? Is he upset and needs a bit of quiet time with you before you deal with the problem? Talk with him about how he feels and what other things he might try. Listen as well. If there needs to be a consequence for what he has done, try to make it both short and suitable. For example, if he is playing with his milk and it spills he could help clean it up.

If something goes wrong it usually means he needs your help. Therefore, punishments which separate him from you are not as useful as keeping him with you for a while, to give him time and space to cool down, and then to help him work out what he can do to make things better.

Discipline is learned in relationships, so if you have an ongoing problem with a child go back first to re-connecting, making sure he feels that your relationship with him is nurturing and supportive.

Toilet training

Your 3-year-old should be capable of all the actions involved in going to the toilet – knowing when his bladder is full, telling you, getting his pants down and up and being able to do wee in the toilet. Most children are toilet trained by the end of this year unless they have been unwell or have got into a battle about it. There will still be accidents when your 3-year-old is too busy doing something until it is too late. It works best to just treat accidents as bad luck and remind him next time when he is very busy. Keeping bad feelings such as shame out of it will help him in the long run. Being dry at night often takes a bit longer – a good time to trial not using the night nappy is when he has been waking up dry in the morning for a couple of weeks.

ICT – Information and Communications Technology

We live in a world where technology is part of almost everything we do – household equipment, cars, TV, digital cameras, phones and so on. Whether or not you have a computer in your home, your child will be working with one when he goes to school and young children can benefit from becoming familiar with them if they have the opportunity.[19] Preschool children and younger, can, for example, practise hand control and hand–eye coordination, become familiar with letters and numbers and how to use a keyboard. They enjoy age-appropriate games and become confident in using basic computer skills. If you decide to let your child use a computer here are some guidelines to consider:

- Use the computer with your child at first and set up easy links to programs suited to his age and interests
- Set up parental controls and Safe Search so that children cannot accidentally find inappropriate content
- Make sure your child uses good posture because his bones are growing and sitting hunched over a computer is not helpful
- Make sure that he has a balance of screen and computer time with plenty of time each day for creative and outdoor play.

For more information about how to introduce children to computers you can download a free booklet called Digital Parenting from <http://parents.vodafone.com> or access the 'Cybersafety' Parent Easy Guide at <www.parenting.sa.gov.au/pegs>.

Resilience

Resilience is the ability to cope with troubles and problems and still get on with living successfully. Research has shown that for children who have a tough start in life, there are some who do well, and these children have the qualities that make up resilience.[20] The qualities that build resilience are in three areas that parents and other adults can encourage: **I can, I have** and **I am**.

I can is about your 3-year-old feeling capable and able to do things in his own life. For this he needs opportunities to try things for himself, encouragement without you taking over, and praise when he does something well. Watch that the things he tries are not too hard for him, leading to disappointment, or too easy. Praise should be for real achievement, not simply for everything he does, so that he feels really capable when he does well. For example, 'I can see that you have got all your buttons done up by yourself, that must have been hard, well done.' As they grow older, children can benefit from learning something they enjoy such as music, craft or sport.

Ali climbed up a rock in a park and was very proud of himself. He asked his dad to watch what he could do. In his enthusiasm he chose to climb a part of the rock that was much too steep for him. His dad let him have a go but Ali fell back down and scraped his legs. He immediately went to try again. His dad then intervened and suggested a more achievable, although still difficult slope. Ali managed to climb this and felt very proud of his success.

> *Young children develop courage from overcoming difficult challenges. Ali had courage because he tried again even after he fell. But young children cannot assess risks. Adults need to assess risks for them – both risks of injury and risks of discouragement from too many failures.*

I have is about your 3-year-old having people around him that he knows he can trust to look after and care for him. This means people whom your child knows he can go to for help, who will not frighten or hurt him if he does something wrong and who enjoy having fun with him. It means knowing how his parents and other people will react and not being scared that one minute they will be loving and the next angry. Of course parents don't have to be perfect, so if you have a bad day be open about it with your child when you say 'sorry' and make up. He also needs some other adults he feels good with: grandparents or other relatives, close friends, a baby sitter or carer and teachers. Being part of a child-friendly community is part of 'I have'. 'I have' is also about being part of continuity, knowing where you come from and where you belong. So take your 3-year-old to family celebrations and visits to the cemetery and tell him stories about his family history and when daddy and mummy were children. Keep photos of your family life and look at the albums together.

Family rituals, the special ways of doing things that belong to your family, also help build resilience. For example, in one family scattered across the country, a ritual developed to play 'Happy Birthday' over the telephone with banging on saucepans as the accompaniment. The ritual says you are special and is part of this family's special way of celebrating birthdays and even the adults look forward to it.

I am is about how your 3-year-old feels about himself. Children need to feel lovable as well as loved. Young children are very sensitive to what you say about them and to them. You show that they are lovable by enjoying spending time with them, by choosing to do things with them, by listening with interest when they talk to you and by showing that you are proud of them. If your 3-year-old boy is afraid to do something and you say 'That is a big thing to try, I bet you can do it' or 'Would you like me to do it with you first?' it shows that you believe in him. If you say 'I give up, you're just a wuss' your child will probably believe you. Letting children help you with what you are doing, or, even better, asking them for help says that you need and value them. If possible make some special time, even if it is short, for each child, each day – time when you just do what they enjoy.

Four-year-old Kelly wanted to take some biscuits to share at pre-school. So, after dinner, Kelly and her 3-year-old sister Sophie helped their mother make biscuits. In their enthusiasm for mixing and stirring and rolling, a coating of flour ended up on both children and the floor. The biscuits survived but their mother thought about how much easier it would have been to put the children to bed and then make the biscuits!

*However she also thought about what the children had learned – that they could help make successful biscuits (**I can**), they could enjoy a shared activity (**I have**), some things about measuring and counting (**I can**), that their mother wanted to spend the time with them (**I am**), and that they could make something to share with others at preschool (**I can, I have**).*

At the core of resilience is a sense of belonging.

> 'Resilience rests fundamentally on relationships. The desire to belong is a basic human need and positive connections with others lie at the very core of psychological development; strong, supportive relationships are critical for achieving and sustaining resilient adaptation'.[21]

You can read more about promoting resilience in children at: <http://resilnet.uiuc.edu/library/grotb95b.html>.

Spirituality

Studies of people who have resilience and cope well with adversity (that is when things go wrong) show that belief in a greater being and/or belonging to a religion help them to cope with hard times.[22,23] So whatever your own spiritual beliefs, you might want to consider giving your child this opportunity. Spirituality involves the search for the meaning of life – why we exist, what our life is for, what happens when we die – as well as a sense of awe and wonder at the greatness of the universe and the beauty of nature. Spirituality also involves values about caring for other people, hope and faith.

Some ways that you can nurture your child's spirituality:

- Take part and involve them in a religious group if you have one. Or look for one that involves children and fits with your own values so your child can take part.
- Read and tell stories about the origins of (your) religion and the origins of the world. These 'mythological' stories are important to making meaning.

- Teach your child a simple prayer to use every day and when they feel alone, thankful or in awe. You can find words in many books, or make up your own.
- Sing simple spiritual songs.
- Rituals are activities that have special meaning. Big rituals are weddings, baptisms and funerals. You can do small rituals with your child such as lighting a candle for someone in a place of worship or in your home.
- There are great religious festivals and children need to experience them, not just watch, so involve your 3-year-old in those that include children. In the Christian tradition these could be Christmas and Easter, and there are many others in the different traditions that make up our culture such as the birthday of Buddha, and Eid ul-Fitr.
- Let your child see the spirituality of special places – the countryside, the sea and places of worship – and be thankful for these gifts to their life.
- Teach your child about the values of caring for others, giving and sharing.

Overview – Three to Four

As we have seen, it is usually very enjoyable to have a 3-year-old. He is able to take a real part in conversations, is easy to be with, and easy to leave with someone else. He is capable of doing most personal things, such as washing and dressing himself with a bit of help and checking. He is trusting, affectionate and lovable. He loves to play with other children, taking turns and sharing (most of the time), and learning about the things he needs to know to get on well with them. However, he is still not very old and there are times when things get too much for him and he needs your help, support and cuddles.

The skills below are ones that your 3-year-old will develop during the year. When and how he learns these things depend not only on his natural ability but very much on the opportunities he has had to try things, and practise them, and what he likes to do. Use the list as a guide and if you have any worries talk with your early childhood teacher and/or a health professional.

Physical development

▶ good physical skills and balance
▶ walks along a plank
▶ jumps off things
▶ dresses himself with a little help
▶ pedals a tricycle
▶ rides a scooter
▶ climbs stairs using alternate feet
▶ throws and catches a big ball
▶ cuts with scissors
▶ holds a pencil correctly.

Social/emotional development

▶ shares and takes turns at least some of the time
▶ likes to play with others of the same age
▶ often chooses playmates because they are doing something he likes to do
▶ has confidence to spend daytime away from main carers
▶ affectionate and friendly
▶ wants to please adults.

Speech and language

▶ speaks clearly so people who don't know him can understand him
▶ may have trouble with some sounds e.g. *ch, l, r, s, sh, th, v, y,* and *z*
▶ knows 1000 or more words
▶ loves stories, rhymes, jokes and songs
▶ learning about the importance of print in his life.

Thinking and learning

▶ knows that his mind is separate and others don't know what he is thinking
▶ knows that objects are not alive and cannot hurt people
▶ can copy a circle, vertical and horizontal lines
▶ draws a very rough person – usually just head and stick legs
▶ can count five or more things
▶ can sort by shape and colour
▶ knows own name and age.

Toys for 3-year-olds

> **Note:** Watch toys for small parts or batteries that could be swallowed.

▶ balls to throw and catch and large bats to hit a ball
▶ scooter with helmet
▶ tricycle with helmet
▶ small two-wheel bike without pedals to push along with feet
▶ dress-ups
▶ cardboard boxes, glue, blunt-ended scissors, old magazines and cards for making things
▶ jigsaw puzzles
▶ DVDs appropriate for their age
▶ books
▶ DUPLO® sets or similar
▶ wooden block sets
▶ toy wagon to pull along and carry toys
▶ sandpit with digging, pouring toys
▶ small garden patch
▶ dolls and prams
▶ toys to take apart and put together
▶ torch
▶ lots of paper to draw on with paint, textas, crayons and pencils
▶ clay or playdough
▶ finger and hand puppets
▶ toy cars, trucks, planes
▶ cubby house.

Chapter 5
Four to Five

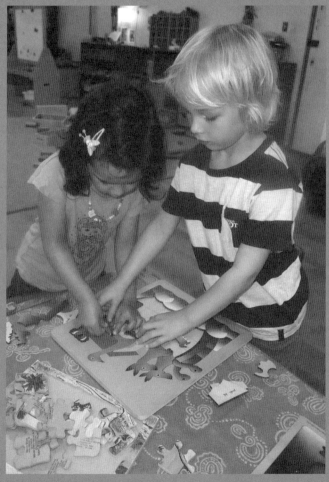

Co-operative play

Your 4-year-old is growing in confidence every day. She is exploring her physical skills, really enjoying playmates and trying out her independence as much as you will allow. Four-year-olds can be full of exuberance; this is somewhat challenging for parents as you don't want to stop their enjoyment of life, but you need to help them to learn what behaviour is OK and what is not. Most 4-year-olds are likely to be in some form of preschool education for part of their week which gives them invaluable learning about social skills, working cooperatively and moving into the big world.

Physical development

Four-year-olds have all the basic physical skills: they can run, jump (including jump over objects), hop a bit, climb, balance and carry things with ease. Some are beginning to skip. They can ride a tricycle and scooter well and may be trying out a bicycle with trainer wheels. They still need parents around to supervise so that they don't take too many risks with climbing and jumping, and to give encouragement to those who are not so daring. They can make quite complicated buildings with wooden blocks or plastic blocks such as DUPLO®.

Four-year-olds are gaining good hand control and can hold scissors properly, hold their pencil well and colour their drawings more or less between the lines. Your 4-year-old can copy a cross and make some marks on paper that look like letters and which she calls writing. She may be able to write the first letter of her name.

You can help your child's hand control by giving her craft and drawing materials to cut, draw and glue. She will manage large pieces best – old magazines as well as Christmas and birthday cards with pictures work well. She will also like large buttons to thread on cord and blocks to build and balance. Outdoors, she enjoys trying new playgrounds, especially adventure-type playgrounds that allow her to use her imagination as well as physical skills. She gets a lot of benefit from throwing and catching balls with you or hitting a ball with a large bat.

Four-year-olds grow more slowly than they did when they were babies and toddlers and they lose some of their early chubbiness as they move from babyhood into childhood.

Social and emotional development

Four-year-olds are social beings. They are beginning to enter the world of real friendships, although at this age the friend is often still someone who happens to be with her and wants to play the same game. You can help by giving her lots of opportunities to play with other children. She will develop even more confidence as she practises playing with friends and going on visits.

Four-year-olds can seem to be 'bossy' and may need some coaching about listening to what others want, but they are also learning to recognise and respond to other children's feelings. When there is a disagreement, it is helpful for parents to talk about both children's feelings as you look for a way forward, helping them to learn the skills that are crucial to social relationships.

Your 4-year-old has developed confidence and trust and is probably happy spending time away from her main carers, either at a friend's house or preschool or on an excursion, unless she has had a distressing experience of separation in the past.

While she is getting better at managing feelings, she is still sensitive to criticism and your good opinion of her. She is often so full-on about trying everything at top pace that she can get overtired and have the occasional tantrum where her feelings 'boil over', just as used to happen when she was 2.

Four-year-olds really want to please you. If she has done something she thinks you won't like, in order to please you she may tell you she did not do it, even when you can clearly see that she did. She has yet to learn that telling the truth is as important to you as doing the right thing. In fact, 4-year-olds still need some help in learning about what is fact and what is a story, what is real and what is not real. All this is teaching time. Rather than try to force her to admit she did not tell the truth, you might just let her know what you saw in a matter-of-fact way, and explain what you would like her to do next time.

Four-year-olds understand more about dangers and can be afraid of the dark or burglars or many other things they hear about. Listen to their fears and reassure them but let them take their own time in facing fears if possible. Reading stories about children or animals who face fears can be helpful. Let them know that you have faith in their ability to overcome their fears. Supporting them to deal with fears at their own pace builds confidence much better than forcing them into situations they are afraid of.

Speech and language

Your 4-year-old can speak clearly and loves to have long and complicated conversations as she develops her language skills. Some may still have troubles with a few sounds such as 's' and 'r'.

They have wide interests and want to know everything about anything that interests them so they may ask questions such as 'Why does the moon come up at night and the sun in the day?' or 'What is sand made of?' If you don't know the answer, take the question seriously and look up the answer or consult someone. This helps your 4-year-old both with her knowledge and because she sees that you consider it important to find out about things.

She likes to find out the meaning of, and to use, long and difficult words as well as tell funny stories and jokes. She may find out about swear words and think these and bathroom words are very funny. I once drove some 4-year-olds on an excursion and they sat in the back of the car saying to each other 'you're a toilet' and bursting into gales of laughter. Four-year-olds are very quick to pick up on what makes parents laugh and then to use those words, often at the wrong time.

Sometimes you can divert them from using an inappropriate word by making up a word that is meaningless but sounds funny for them to use instead. Sometimes you just need to say that you do not like to hear that word and you will not respond if they say it. Most 4-year-olds give up on saying something if they get no response.

Continue to read stories to her every day and sometimes ask questions about the story, such as what she thinks might happen, why she likes a story and which characters she likes. Point out stop and speed signs as you approach them. She might like to look out for signs and remind you what to do. If you sing an alphabet song she will learn the letters and might be able to pick out some letters, such as those in her own name, when she sees them in shops and magazines. If you show her she will be able to recognise her name in print, and may learn to write it. If she has different things to do on different days you could make a picture calendar with the name of the day written at the top and pictures to represent the various activities.

Thinking and learning

Your 4-year-old is putting together a lot of the things she has been learning about over the past three years. She uses symbolism (where something stands for something else) a lot more than she used to in her play, and she plays quite complicated symbolic games. Her bedroom or cubby house may be a fairy dell one day, a forest the next, and a pirate ship on another day.

She understands what is real and what is not real, such as when you explain that some of the things shown on TV are not real, although it will still be several more years before she really starts to question Father Christmas and the tooth fairy.

Her memory is improving too and with help she can tell you what she did last week or while on holiday, as well as what happened yesterday.

She can count up to about 20 and really understand what numbers up to three mean, so she can look at cups on the table and say 'there are two cups'. She sorts things by size, shape and colour or what group they are – for example, animals – although she may still make some mistakes. She is also improving her noticing skills so that her drawings have much more detail in them.

Talk about things like yesterday and tomorrow; let her try pouring her glass of milk or water; sort toys into categories such as blocks, pencils, toy cars as she puts them away; talk about bigger and smaller, slower and faster, longer and shorter, so she can use these words and compare different things. She is not able to tell the time yet but you can talk about what time it is that you do various things and point to it on the clock.

Many 4-year-olds enjoy puzzles – make sure that they are challenging enough but not too hard – and simple problem-solving computer games. If you borrow some puzzles from a toy library, as she learns to solve them you can regularly borrow new ones to try.

Go for walks around your area and get her to notice landmarks and find the way home.

Children learn best from doing what they enjoy so follow their lead and take opportunities for teaching, but don't make life a lesson!

Play

Four-year-olds are keen to explore their physical boundaries and enjoy outdoor adventures such as playgrounds, bush walks, ball games and trips to the beach. They are starting to explore the world of friends and playing together, especially including symbolic and imaginary games. Sometimes these games continue over time; sometimes they may finish quickly when the players each want to do something different and haven't yet learned how to negotiate who does what.

Play-based learning

Play involves activities where children choose what to do and how to do it. During play, children are motivated because they choose and they have fun. Most of their other activities are organised and guided by adults. In play, adults provide time, space and materials, and join in when the child invites them, but children lead the play.

Play is the way children learn, as well as the way they relax and have fun so play at home is important. Much of what they need to know in their education and in living is better learned through active participation than through sitting and listening. Everyone learns best through doing. Play helps children work through problems and gain a sense of control in situations where they feel powerless, and build strong relationships.[24]

Some examples of the value of play as a learning experience are in Table 5.1.

Table 5.1. The value of play as a learning experience

Cognitive – Thinking Skills	Physical – Motor Skills
e.g. planning, problem solving, counting, making patterns, matching, reasoning, measuring, predicting	e.g. coordination, strength, small and large muscle development, balance
<ul><li>Games with rules</li><li>Pretend games</li><li>Stories</li><li>Puzzles</li><li>Painting and drawing</li><li>Collecting things</li></ul>	<ul><li>Ball play</li><li>Riding toys</li><li>Making things</li><li>Painting and drawing</li><li>Mosaics</li><li>Threading</li></ul>
Social/Emotional Skills	**Literacy and Language – Reading, Writing, Talking, Listening, Creating and Viewing**
e.g. friendship skills, managing feelings, empathy, resolving conflicts	
<ul><li>Play with other children</li><li>Role play – mothers and fathers, careers</li><li>Superhero/fairy play</li><li>Hide and seek/peek-a-boo games</li><li>Adventure play</li><li>Dramatic play</li></ul>	<ul><li>Reading and telling stories</li><li>Songs and rhymes</li><li>Play with other children</li><li>Making up games</li><li>Dramatic play</li><li>Drawing and writing</li></ul>

Much of the learning values of play includes learning in many areas, not just one. For example, playing mothers and fathers involves social skills, planning skills, communication and language and physical activity.

Play is also an important part of early childhood education, including the first years of school. Sometimes parents whose children have started preschool wonder why there is so much play – 'after all they can do that at home'. As we can see from the above examples, play develops all the skills that are part of early education and research has shown that play-based learning in young children is very effective in skill development.[25]

Early childhood educators are skilled in understanding what children need for their education and how play contributes to this.[26]

They:
- plan play environments
- provide appropriate materials for the different learning areas
- help children to extend their interests in constructive ways
- assess learning and developmental strengths and challenges and provide activities to support these
- provide support for individual and group play
- assist children with social skill development in group play
- encourage curiosity, perseverance and motivation.

Sexual development

Four-year-olds are interested in bodies – their own and those of others. They may want to look at each other's bodies, checking out similarities and differences. They are interested in how babies come, what happens in bathrooms and have many questions about topics like these. If you answer questions honestly, simply and naturally, without going into more detail than they ask for, you open the way for them to be able to tell you anything that worries them. Also talk to them about how some parts of their bodies are private. Depending on the situation you might simply say, 'Your penis is private so we keep it covered', or 'We don't touch other people's private parts'. They may masturbate, for comfort or because it feels good. It is not helpful to make your child feel guilty about this but remind her that it is something she should only do in private. As with younger children, if your child masturbates a lot it may be because there is something worrying her that needs your attention. If your 4-year-old talks about sex, or asks questions that show knowledge beyond other children of her age, check with a health professional, as it is possible that someone has been talking or acting inappropriately with her.

Some other things to know about 4- to 5-year-olds

Behaviour

Four-year-olds are full of energy and their behaviour is often very boisterous, sometimes 'over the top'.

Your 4-year-old uses her imagination to make up stories that turn into rowdy games. She can become very excited, using words meant to shock you and generally gets carried away. She needs a watchful eye to be sure she doesn't get into danger. She needs you to appreciate her energy and join in and enjoy her sense of fun, while also setting limits about consideration for others, helping to clean up her own mess, and taking a break to do quiet activities if things are getting out of hand.

Discipline

Discipline is about teaching. You teach your child what she needs to know to get on in the world and to be safe. Some starting points for effective teaching are:

- Make sure your relationship with your child is good – spend time listening to her and being with her
- Make sure she knows clearly what you expect her to do
- Don't expect her to be able to manage rules on her own; she needs you to be watching over her and helping her when needed
- Give her choices where possible e.g. 'Do you want to throw the ball outside or play with your blocks in here?'

- Make consequences simple and relevant e.g. 'The blocks have to be picked up before you get out any more toys. Would you like some help?'
- Plan for difficult times e.g. late in the day when you are busy and your child is tired
- Keep a child who is not able to manage her behaviour with you for a while – she needs your help
- Provide relaxing activities for an overstressed child – something to eat, a story, a bath, a walk outside
- When necessary, have a consequence which helps your child make up for what she has done
- Teaching, positive discipline and monitoring your child (i.e. knowing what she is doing) paves the way for good learning.
- After problems, always reconnect.

Daniel's older sister Mia was sitting at the kitchen table doing her homework. Daniel took a wet cloth and smeared Mia's picture. 'Don't do that' said Daniel's mother as she prepared the dinner, 'go and play with your blocks'. She took the cloth away from him. A few minutes later Daniel smeared the picture again. His mother was angry, Mia was upset and so was Daniel. Later Daniel's mother thought about what had happened and made a plan. The next night she had some 'homework' for Daniel: a paper and pencils to make a drawing of his day. Both children did their homework side by side while the dinner was cooked.

When problems with children recur, parents may be able to think about what each child's needs are and make a plan to prevent the problem happening.

Keep in mind that they learn much more from what you do, than from what you tell them to do!

Toilet training

Your 4-year-old is probably fully toilet trained during the day and can manage her own toilet needs, although she still may need help with the toilet paper from time to time. She can hold on longer before going to the toilet and should be remembering to wash her hands afterwards.

She is likely to have occasional accidents as she gets involved in play and forgets about her bladder; then there is a last minute rush which is sometimes too late. If you can see this is likely to happen a gentle reminder is in order. Your child may say she doesn't need to go, so you might have to insist and offer to mind her game for her while she is gone. If she does have an accident, try to be philosophical about it. There will probably be more in the next couple of years.

Many 4-year-olds are dry at night but some, especially boys, take up to a few more years before they achieve this. Bedwetting is not the child's fault, it is just the way they grow and often runs in families. Star charts and other rewards are not likely to work because the child is not in control of it, although sometimes they work for a couple of nights as the child is tense or excited and sleeps more lightly. If you ignore it and don't let your child be upset, she will grow out of bedwetting in her own time. If a child who is toilet trained at night or day starts to wet again, it is a good idea to check with your doctor. Sometimes it can be due to a health problem.

Superheroes

Parents are sometimes concerned whether children should be allowed to play at being superheroes such as Spiderman or Buzz Lightyear. Even if it doesn't always seem so, children are fairly powerless in their worlds; they are often being told what they can and can't do, what to do now, or stop doing now and so on. Playing about superheroes or fairies can give them a sense of being powerful which helps compensate for this. The arguments against superhero play is that the roles are stereotyped; they don't encourage creative play; they can encourage rough and aggressive play. The difficulty with banning it is that it is likely to go 'underground' and become more important to children because it is banned.

There are ways you can make superhero play more acceptable. You can make sure that there are some parts of your play space where superheroes are not allowed and where quieter children can play in peace. You can make rules about what they are allowed to do, for example, not hurt people or things. You can also talk with your child about what the superheroes do – mostly they are a force for good, rescuing people in trouble and defeating the bad guys. And talk about how the people who are getting 'zapped' with various ray guns might feel, and what else the superhero could do to win the war against evil. All of this helps to counter the stereotype and encourage children to play more imaginatively.

Attention seeking

Visitors are admiring cute 1-year-old Sofia. Four-year-old Manuel begins to dance around and 'show off', saying 'Look at me, look at me'. His embarrassed mother says 'Stop that silly behaviour, Manuel.' One of the visitors says, 'It's just attention seeking'.

Manuel is feeling left out and needing to feel that he matters too. His actions get him the wrong sort of attention. Young children don't know how to communicate what they need and their attempts often lead to getting into trouble, rather than the love they are seeking. It is hard to always give what they need but if parents are aware that what is called 'attention seeking' is really the child's need to reconnect, they can respond to the need, not the behaviour (or both if necessary). Mum might say 'Here is my special big boy. Come over here and have a hug, Manuel'.

Overview – Four to Five

This has probably been the last full year for your child to be at home and in some ways still your baby. Your 4-year-old loves to get away and do her own thing, yet still at times wants to be cuddled or helped as things get too much for her. Four-year-olds have grown out of toddlerhood and grown in confidence. They are often exuberant, excitable and noisy. They like to show off what they can do and try out toilet words to their own great amusement. They are learning to play well with other children when the game suits them and to relate to other children's feelings.

Every child is different and has different experiences that affect their growing and learning. Use the list below as a general guide only.

Physical development
▶ physically capable: run, jump, hop a bit, climb, balance and carry things with ease
▶ beginning to skip
▶ likely to take risks with climbing and jumping
▶ can ride a tricycle
▶ rides a scooter well
▶ good hand control and can hold scissors properly for cutting
▶ holds and controls a pencil well
▶ makes complicated structures with wooden or plastic blocks.

Social/emotional development
▶ learning to recognise and respond to other children's feelings
▶ can be 'bossy'
▶ more independent

▶ sensitive to criticism and your good opinion

▶ can get overtired and have the occasional tantrum

▶ loves to play with other children

▶ still needs your help in learning about what is real and what is not real

▶ understands more about dangers and can be afraid of things on TV.

Speech and language

▶ speaks clearly and loves talking

▶ may still have trouble with a few sounds

▶ curious and asks many questions

▶ interest in new words

▶ likes to tell funny stories and jokes

▶ finds out about swear words and toilet words and may think these are funny

▶ can read own name and may be able to write it

▶ recognises some letters and numbers.

Thinking and learning

▶ enjoys symbolic play and often plays involved symbolic games

▶ memory is improving – can tell you what they did last week or on holiday as well as yesterday

▶ can count up to about 20

▶ sorts things by size, shape and colour or what group they are

▶ talks about things like yesterday and tomorrow

▶ enjoys puzzles and can do quite complex jigsaws.

Toys for 4-year-olds

Note: Watch toys for small parts or batteries that could be swallowed.

▶ tricycles or two-wheeled bike with trainers
▶ scooters
▶ wagon to load up
▶ dress-ups
▶ tent or playhouse
▶ dolls and dollhouse
▶ cars and trucks
▶ puppets
▶ jigsaw puzzles
▶ DUPLO® blocks or LEGO®, depending on finger control for small blocks
▶ books
▶ preschool computer games
▶ suitable DVDs
▶ pencils, crayons, paper, paint, glue and scissors
▶ balls and bats.

Chapter 6

Five to Six

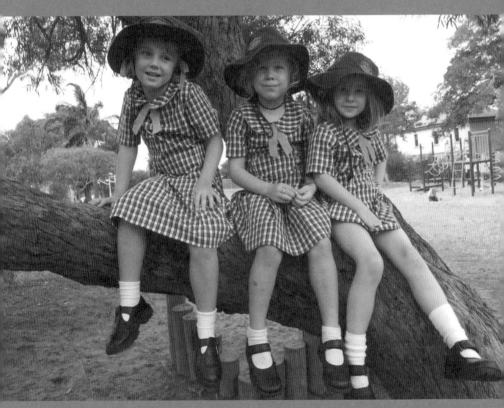

Starting school – it helps to have friends

Five to 6 is a big year for children. Some time during this year most children start school. This means moving away from the comfortable world of family, home and carers into the big world of children. For most children it is both exciting and stressful. Studies have shown that children's stress level goes up in the months before they start school as well as at the time of transition to school[27], so even thinking about starting school is a very big event in their lives. The exuberant, boisterous 4-year-old is now the youngest and smallest in the schoolyard with many new expectations of him – how to behave in the classroom and schoolyard as well as new learning. The challenges are exciting and being a school person gives your child a sense of pride and lots of new experiences.

Physical development

Five-year-olds are active, adventurous people. They climb trees, climb to the top of playground equipment, and may ride a scooter or a two-wheeler bike with training wheels. They are starting to skip and may want to try skipping with a rope. They can stand on one foot for a short time. They can throw and catch a ball as long as it is not too small; practising ball skills will be helpful to them later on as they play sport that involves balls. They can also hit a ball with a bat. They can dress themselves, attend to their toilet needs, put shoes on the correct feet and use eating tools well.

Your child has good hand control, can cut fairly accurately and colour in his drawings, keeping between the lines. His drawings are much more detailed and drawings of people may include things like eyebrows as well as eyes, ears, hair and hands. He is able to copy some letters and will have a well-established preference for one hand.

Physical exercise and good balance that come from riding a bike and walking along a wall also help thinking and learning.

Social and emotional development

Five-year-olds are usually fairly settled and easy to get along with. They are willing to share toys and take turns with other children. Playing with friends is very important to them as they develop the skills of being a friend, such as considering others, sometimes playing what the other child chooses, and being sympathetic if someone is hurt. They can better manage their feelings, and talk about problems and how to solve them rather than just react.

There are many new challenges in moving into the world of school. These include making friends and learning to play in a group, as well as managing in the schoolyard at lunch time with minimal adult support. Your child needs lots of confidence to manage these challenges and your support and belief in him is really important. Although he is developing independence in many ways, parents are still the centre of his security and wellbeing and he needs your support as much as ever as he moves further out into the big world.

Often 5-year-olds come home from school physically and emotionally exhausted. Your child may need some non-pressured time and space to relax when he first gets home. He may not want to answer questions about the day or take up other activities until he has had a break and a snack. If both parents are working most of the time you might not have the energy to give a lot of support, so it is important to try to get a balance in your own lives in order to give children what they need.

Speech and language

Five-year-olds can usually speak clearly and confidently and use correct grammar. You can help your child by having conversations with him, explaining any words he doesn't know, and using interesting words and ideas yourself. If he asks you about things you don't know, show him how you look it up. Encourage him to ask. This helps him learn to solve problems.

> Nathan (age 5): 'She started it.'
>
> Julie (age 6): 'He escalated it.'
>
> Nathan: 'She started it and escalated it.'
>
> *Nathan and Julie are both showing their interest in new words. They are also competing for their parent's attention and approval (see Sibling rivalry, pages 130–31).*

Your 5-year-old should be able to tell you his name and age and be learning his address. If you have not taught him his address, now is a good time. He may also be able to tell you when his birthday is.

He is interested in longer stories and in talking to you about what is happening in the story and what he thinks might happen next. Reading stories is one of the best things you can do to help your child to want to learn to read. You might want to join a library with a children's section where there are lots of books your child can choose from. Once he is at school there will be books from school as well. Allow him to choose stories that he likes, and let him see how the words tell the story that the picture is about. Tell stories about what you did when you were a child; these are unfailingly interesting to children, especially funny stories. Five-year-olds love jokes and simple riddles, although often their jokes seem to be known only to themselves. Bedtime is a relaxing time to have stories, snuggle up and end the day feeling good.

Knowing the alphabet and recognising some letters and numbers will help your child feel more comfortable when he starts school. Giving him lessons might put him off but you can play games that show him that language is important. When you are driving you could look for cars with a five in the number plate (because he is 5), let him help you select your favourite brands in shops, and help him write his name on his drawings and his special drawer. You can make a game of noticing signs on lifts, doors and buildings, labels on packets and street directions if he is interested.

Some 5-year-olds still have difficulty with saying a few sounds, but your child should be easy to understand. If people who don't know him well cannot easily understand him it is worth checking with a health professional.

The most important thing is to really listen when your child is talking to you. Make sure you show you are listening by your reply.

Thinking and learning

Your child now has a much better understanding of time and by the end of the year may be able to tell the time on the hour and what day of the week it is. He can talk meaningfully about yesterday and tomorrow.

> Calen was having a friend over to play in two days' time. Calen asked, 'It is tomorrow, tomorrow?' His father said, 'Yes, it is the day after tomorrow'.
>
> *Calen is learning to understand about time in a practical way by counting tomorrows. His father is helping by giving 'tomorrow tomorrow' a name.*

He can sort things by size and shape and colour or type – for example, he could put all the red cows together. You can help by giving him things to sort for you and by helping him see how things fit into groups, such as cows and horses are animals, carrot and broccoli are vegetables. He can count at least 20 objects. By the end of the year he can work out what numbers go together to make 10.

> Grandad was reading a story about a sloth. 'Are sloths herbivores or carnivores?' asked Noah. Grandad did not know so they looked it up on the internet and found that sloths eat small insects and leaves. 'Well they must be omnivores,' said Noah.
>
> *Noah is learning about classifying things in different ways. He knows that sloths are animals and he has now put them into another group according to what they eat.*

Most children like to play some board and card games with you. Start with simple ones, such as Snap and UNO®. Make sure he has a good chance to win so he does not get discouraged.

Your child develops confidence in being able to do things for himself by practising doing things and managing them: puzzles that are not too hard or too easy (5-year-olds can do puzzles with quite a large number of pieces, although sometimes they may get bored with a big puzzle), simple tasks to help you, making a picture by drawing, colouring, cutting and sticking, and cooking with your support. When he comes to you with a problem, talk with him about how to solve it, encouraging him to try his own ideas.

Some computer time, if you have one at home, can help children with thinking and language skills and develop confidence as well as provide enjoyment. Free interactive websites that children enjoy exploring help them with many of the skills they need to learn. (For suggestions see 'Websites for school beginners and upwards' on page 195.)

Once they start school, children need lots of time to do the things they are good at and enjoy, so they are not just practising the things they need to improve.

Learning something special?

You may be thinking about whether there are any after-school activities that your child would enjoy. A main consideration is to make sure that he has time to play and be with his friends, so that his time is not filled with things he 'has to do'. Five-year-olds are too young for organised sport, but throwing and hitting balls with you in the backyard is good training for any future sport that your child might want to take up. The recommended age for taking part in a junior team, if your child wants to, is 8 years or older.

If he has not learned to swim it is a good time for swimming lessons, if they are not provided by the school.

Apart from these suggestions, you could look out for your child's own particular interests and abilities. If he has something he is good at and enjoys, especially if it is something he can do with friends, it helps him with the hard things he has to do and learn. The confidence he gets from activities he is good at and enjoys carries over into believing in himself and sticking at hard things.

Sometimes you see what your child enjoys and you can encourage him in this and show him that you are proud of what he can do. Or you might try something that his friends are doing and see if he likes it. Often a child finds something he likes at school. There is no rush and children at this age are quite happy simply with school or preschool and play with friends, so if he is not really interested, or it is hard for you to manage, leave it for later on.

Children may start comparing themselves with others and worry about winning and losing. Helping your child to see that everyone is different, and that he can do some special things while his friends do other things well, assists him to learn to appreciate differences.

Play

Five-year-olds enjoy playing with playmates, making up symbolic games where they may be fairies, superheroes, train drivers or families with parents and children. They still need some discreet adult supervision to ensure that no-one is being unfairly treated or left out. This helps them to learn good social skills. If there is no real unfairness or unhappiness they do best if they are allowed to sort out their own problems and difficulties – they learn well that way. If one child is distressed or left out or there is bullying, they need help.

Your 5-year-old loves going to playgrounds and trying out his physical skills on the equipment, playing throwing and catching games, or hitting a tennis ball that you throw to him. Handball is often popular as well as learning to skip with a skipping rope.

He likes board games and card games. He enjoys drawing and painting and likes to have a go at beginning crafts such as mosaics, clay modelling (including painting the model) and cooking.

And of course reading to him is still most important, because he loves it, it is close time with parents, and it helps him to love stories and want to learn to read. It also helps him to think about problem solving and other things that happen in his life as he sees what happens in the stories.

Five-year-olds enjoy movies that are suitable for their age and many are available on DVD. Children's TV is also popular and many 5-year-olds have favourite programs. Your child may need to be reminded that he needs to keep a balance in his life. Time sitting in front of TV is not time when he is getting exercise, getting outside in the fresh air, using his own imagination and play skills, or playing with friends. Some outdoor play every day, when possible, really helps with a good night's sleep, as well as physical fitness.

Sleeping

Children starting school need good sleep. Your child might need reminding that it is time for bed and also some help to relax into sleep. Sitting by your child's bed and reading stories, talking about the day and saying special good nights will help your child relax. There are some relaxation activities you can do if your child wants them or you think he would benefit (see 'Early childhood resources' on page 192). Some children need a light on to sleep and the door to be open or shut, depending on how they feel.

If your child tends to sleep in in the mornings, try getting all of his school things ready the night before so there is not a big rush.

Nightmares are common, where children wake up crying and need your comfort. They can often tell you what the dream was about and you can reassure them. If your child is having a lot of nightmares, there might be too many stresses in his life. If he can't tell you what his worries are, you could talk with his teacher about what is happening at school. Sometimes just saying to a child that you want to help, and it is OK to tell you anything when he wants to, will encourage him to tell you. When children are relaxed at bedtime they often talk about what is on their minds.

Night terrors are different. These happen in the deepest part of sleep and the child has no memory of them, and usually does not wake. You can hold or comfort your child but it is not necessary to try to wake him. The cause of night terrors is not known, although sometimes they happen when a child has a fever. They can be quite distressing but children grow out of them. If your child has them regularly at the same time of night, sometimes gently half-waking him about a quarter of an hour before it happens and then soothing him back to sleep with gentle words may prevent the night terror.

Sexual development

Five-year-olds who have started school are entering a world of older children with more knowledge than they have – some of it correct and some of it not! It is important to have open communication with your child, so he knows he can tell you or ask about anything he is unsure of or that is worrying him. Looking at a book together about how a baby is made is a good way to show that you are open to talk about these things and paves the way for any questions he has. Your child may have questions about same-sex couples or children with two mums or two dads. You can just answer these simply and honestly, saying, for example, that sometimes two mums or two dads love each other and want to have a family of their own, just as your family does.

Five-year-olds sometimes talk about being boyfriends and girlfriends and whom they will marry. This is part of exploring relationships and copying what they see around them, especially on TV. It helps to tell them that they will change as they grow up and probably find someone quite different to be their boyfriend or girlfriend. This helps particularly if their chosen 'spouse' rejects them.

If your 5-year-old picks up sexual language and jokes from school that are offensive, you could explain to him that sex is a natural part of living and that you don't want him to make that kind of joke or use those words. He may say them just to see what you will do. Sometimes, ignoring (once you have explained that you don't like it) helps your child to see that you don't respond to that kind of talk. If he does it when there are other people there, you could take him away from the group and explain that he can't be in the group if he doesn't talk appropriately.

Some other things to know about 5- to 6-year-olds

Bedwetting

Your 5-year-old can manage all his toilet needs well, although some children (about 10 per cent) still wet the bed, sometimes until they are 9 or 10. If your child still wets the bed, or starts to wet the bed again, it is a good idea to have a check-up with your doctor to make sure there is no illness causing it. Usually it is to do with maturation and everyone matures at different rates. Bedwetting tends to run in families and be more common in boys, so you may have a dad or uncle who has had the same problem and can reassure your child that it will go in time. Unless it is very worrying for your child it works well to use special training pants at night and to wait until he grows out of it. Neither punishment nor star charts are likely to work because the bedwetting is not in the child's conscious control. (Sometimes these will work for a couple of days as the child is thinking about it and sleeps more lightly than usual but this does not last.) Treating it as matter-of-factly as you can helps your child to be more relaxed and not feel bad about it. If an overnight sleepover at school comes up, and your child wants to go, let the teacher know. Your child will not be the only one in the class who wets the bed and teachers are accustomed to dealing with it tactfully. Sleepovers are more likely to happen in the next few years than the first year at school however. If he wants to sleep over at a friend's place, you could discuss it with the friend's mother to see if it could be worked out so that your child is not embarrassed. If not, have friends to your place for sleepovers instead.

Telling the truth

By about 3 years, children have realised that you can't read their minds – they have their own thoughts. This is when they begin to make up stories and parents help them by talking to them about what are stories, what are wishes and what is real. Your five-year-old knows that some things he does make you unhappy or cross, and he wants to please you more than he wants to tell the truth. So he may say that he did not do something that he clearly did. You can help by letting him know that you will be really pleased if he always tells you the truth, even when he does something wrong. It also helps not to put him on the spot, when you know he did something. Rather than ask him if he did it, you could say, 'I see you knocked over the glass and it spilt on the carpet. I'll help you get a cloth to wipe it up'.

Starting school

Before your child starts school, help him to get to know some other children beginning at the same school if possible. Have them over to play so that your child has some children that he knows from the start. Friends make a big difference to a happy beginning at school. Having one special friend can be a problem – it is better to encourage your child to have several playmates (one at a time for play dates usually works best at first) so that if there is a falling out your child has others to play with. If you see that your child is having difficulty joining a group or with a friend, you may be able to give him some gentle coaching about things like smiling and being friendly, joining in rather than pushing in, and taking turns.

Check with the school before starting day about what things your child needs to know and wear and take to school so he is not worried about having the right things. Make sure he has clothes that he can deal with easily when going to the toilet and that he can open his lunch and manage his backpack. One or more trips to the school (walking if it is close enough) when the time gets near will show him where it is in relation to your home, which helps him feel more secure. You may also be able to show him where the toilets are and where you will wait for him each day.

Don't expect much of your child at the end of the school day. He may come home grumpy and tired and need some space before he is ready to play happily. Don't worry if he shares his lunch with others or does not eat it all; children are often too excited to eat a good lunch. Having something for him to eat when he gets home, or in the car if you have to do shopping, will help and so will an early dinner. If you are concerned about how your child is getting on in the classroom or the schoolyard, try not to show it by asking a lot of questions. Children very quickly pick up on parents' concerns and become more worried or do not want to tell you. So if you don't get an answer to 'What was the best thing about your day?' leave it for a while. Children will tell you in their own time.

Your child might ask if he can take a special toy to school to show the other children. He needs to be aware that there is a real risk that the toy may be lost or broken as teachers are unable to keep a watch on toys all the time. Talk with him about what he might choose to take that is not too special if he really wants to take something, and have a friend over to play with the special toy at another time.

Learning at home (Homework)

Some schools give some work to take home from the first year of school. If your child has homework you need to show you think it is important and support him in doing it. The homework might be quite challenging at first, so having your help will give your child a feeling of confidence that he can cope and a much more positive start to his school days.

If your child has homework to do, try to find a time when he is relaxed: not straight after school, but not when he is tired or rushed. He needs some time to play at the end of the school day. Because he is new to learning to read, he needs lots of success and encouragement. If he is struggling with a word in his book you can help by suggesting that he looks at the picture: look at the letter that the word starts with and help him sound it out. If he is really not able to work it out you might say it for him; then he can read it after you and be successful. Helping your child to think about the sounds that make up words will help his reading. If he is looking around the room or getting upset, take a break and come back to it later.

Another way that you can help your 5-year-old is by supporting your child's learning of the most commonly used words – sight words – that he needs to be able to recognise. The teacher will have a list of these and they may be a part of your child's homework. It is important that your child gets on top of these first reading challenges and feels successful because learning these early skills starts a lifetime of being able to enjoy reading.

Children need to feel confident at school in order to make the most of it. For this they need parents' help to do the early steps well. What is really important for your child is not only what he knows, but that he is learning how to think about things, how to find things out and how to solve problems for himself.

> **Note:** If you find that supporting your child with homework is not working out, perhaps because one of you is getting very uptight, talk with the teacher about the best way you can be helpful. Learning needs to be something he wants to do.

Separation problems

Sometimes children find it hard to separate from parents when they first go to school, and may say they don't want to go. This is understandable – it is a big world out there. You can help by listening to their feelings and being understanding. Try not to show it if you are worried yourself. Children often misunderstand and think that if a parent is worried there really is something to worry about! Showing your child that you understand how he feels but you have faith that he will be able to manage will help his confidence.

Some things that help

- Try not to be late at pick-up time, or if you have to be late for some reason, let the school know so they can tell your child.
- Read stories about starting new things – 'The Kissing Hand' is one story that often helps.[28]
- Tell your child what you will be doing during the day so he knows where you will be.
- Let him decide how he wants to say goodbye to you.
- Sometimes a child does better if a friend's parent takes him to school and your child says goodbye to you at home.
- As he learns to cope better you can give him encouragement for successes along the way.

If the problem of saying goodbye goes on, think about what could be worrying him. For example, if parents are having lots of arguments children become stressed and may find it hard to separate at school. Sometimes the child is reminded of an earlier separation (e.g. due to illness) which made him sad.

In the long run, children who have separation problems at the start of school usually overcome them and do very well.

Sibling rivalry

Brothers and sisters can be really good friends and supports for each other but there will also be quarrels and times when they don't get on well. The main reason for this is the need for them to share their parents' love. Each child wants to be the chosen one and as much as you love them all, it is not easy for them always to feel this. The other reason is that they are learning about getting along and living with other people – sharing play space, owning and sharing toys, difference in temperaments and, of course, sharing parent time, especially if one child has more needs. This learning will stand them in good stead.

Some ways to help are:

- Make sure each child gets some regular individual time with you.
- Do some fun things together as a family and show your children how to negotiate differences by what you do.
- Help children to understand that being fair does not always mean getting exactly the same, as needs are different at different times.
- Ensure that each child gets some individual space and time to be with their own friends and interests.
- When there is an argument, it is good for them to solve it themselves if possible. If you need to intervene try helping them to work out a solution that works for both of them (e.g. taking turns for a favourite game), rather than just separating them or telling them what to do. Sometimes they need to separate for a short time first in order to cool down, then come back to solving the problem.
- Make sure they know that you will always love them and there will be enough of what they need for each of them.

More resources on this subject are listed in 'Early childhood resources' at the end of this book (page 192).

Fathers

Research shows that fathers are very important to children in the primary school years.[29] Children do better at school when their fathers take an active interest by talking to them about what they are doing, giving a hand if needed, encouraging, going to the school to meet the teacher, helping at working bees and attending when their child is taking part in special activities. Both girls and boys need this support.

If your child doesn't have a father in his or her life, you may have another male relative or friend who could help support your child. Young children are learning what it is like to be a man or a woman and they need to see men and woman showing respect for each other and themselves, and showing them how to act as considerate, caring, assertive human beings.

Overview – Five to Six

You may have had a very exuberant and 'over-the-top' 4-year-old who has now started school and experienced being a small part of a much bigger world. Some people say that the first year of school is one of the hardest years of childhood. Your child may be more fearful than before, need more support and have less confidence. This is partly because of all the new things he is facing and partly because he knows and understands much more of what is going on around him. He can play well with friends, although friendships may still be quite changeable, and he can be hurt by upsets with friends. He can also be very caring of others. He is beginning to understand about competing with others and to care about losing. He is learning about games with rules and cares about fair play.

He is likely to be tired at the end of the day and perhaps grumpy or easily upset. He needs your understanding and support and some extra tolerance as he moves into this new phase of his childhood.

The list below is a general one to give you an idea about what you might expect in this year. However, all children develop differently. If you have any concerns about your child's development, talk with a health professional. You will either get reassurance that your child is doing well, or if there is any problem you will be able to get help for your child.

Physical development
- very able physically – runs fast, climbs well
- may gallop and hop
- stands on one leg for a short time
- pedals a tricycle well
- walks along a line on the ground

- runs up and down stairs using alternate feet on each stair
- bounces a ball (handball)
- throws and catches, and hits balls with a bat
- good hand control – draws detailed pictures and colours within the lines, and does some crafts
- can dress and undress
- manages his own eating, including chopsticks if he has been taught, and toilet needs.

Social/emotional development

- enjoys playing with others
- can be best friends with one child one day and with someone different the next day
- usually joins in group play successfully – may need some help and coaching
- pleasing parents is still most important to him
- may tell untruths if they think that the truth will not please parents
- may have difficulty separating to start school at first
- may lose confidence when they first start school and compare themselves with others.

Speech and language

- good grasp of language and speaks well, using long words and correct parts of speech and can hold a good conversation with adults as well as their friends
- interested in words and the meaning of words
- enjoys telling jokes and simple riddles (sometimes it is hard for adults to 'get the joke')
- knows his name, age and address if he has been told

- speech is clear
- knows more than 2000 words.

Thinking and learning

- understands more about time – today, tomorrow, yesterday;
- may be able to tell what day it is, or what o'clock it is
- sorts objects into collections
- can read many letters and knows the alphabet
- can write some words including own name
- reads and writes three-letter words by the end of the year
- says numbers up to 50
- can count objects up to 20 or so.

Toys for 5-year-olds

- scooter, with helmet
- bicycle with trainer wheels and helmet
- junior tennis racquet and balls
- junior cricket bat and soft balls
- football/basketball
- skipping rope
- craft sets
- paints and books to paint in
- books (school beginners still love to be read to)
- jigsaw puzzles
- craft materials
- simple board and card games
- dress-ups
- LEGO® sets
- dollhouse and/or cubby house.

Chapter 7

Six to Seven

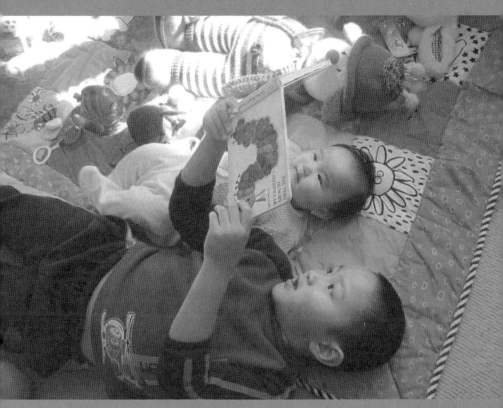

Sharing the enjoyment of reading

Six-year-olds are going into their second year at school – they are no longer the babies of the school. The world outside their home and their friendships with other children are becoming more important. They are meeting lots of new people and comparing what they have learnt at home with what happens at other people's houses and what the teacher says. They are also learning values about what is important and about right and wrong. They may start challenging parents on information but parents are still the most important people in their lives. Many 6-year-olds have some emotional ups and downs. They need parents to help them make sense of all the new experiences they are having and to help them to manage their time so they have a healthy balance between homework, play, friends, family, other activities if they have them, and rest.

Physical development

Six-year-olds are losing their first teeth. Some children may still occasionally wet their pants at school from trying to hold on too long while they are busy doing other things or because it is a bit scary going to the school toilets. Putting a spare pair of pants in the bottom of their backpack for emergencies can be a good idea, as well as letting them know that this happens to lots of children if they do have an 'accident'.

Your 6-year-old's physical skills are good and she runs, jumps, climbs and balances well so she really enjoys climbing and balancing play equipment. She can ride a two-wheeled bike with trainer wheels well. Many 6-year-olds can turn somersaults. She likes to be on the move and cannot easily sit still for long. She may be awkward from time to time; however she is becoming much more coordinated.

Her small muscles are developing and she has good hand control for using pencils and paints, as well as for crafts which need adept finger control and perhaps learning a musical instrument.

Her ball skills such as throwing, catching, hitting and kicking are still developing and as these skills will be important for playing games later on, she will get a lot of benefit from playing with you in the backyard or park.

Six-year-olds usually lead busy and active lives so good sleep is important. Spending some quiet time or reading a story with her before bedtime is a good way to help her relax for the night, as are children's meditations if her day has been stressful. One is provided in the reference list.[30]

Social and emotional development

Six-year-olds compare themselves to others and often find it hard to lose when they play games. If you play games with your child, where she can win at least some of the time, it helps build her confidence. It also helps if you try to avoid too many games where someone wins and someone loses. Help her to think about what she wants to get out of the game, rather than winning. For example, maybe she could work towards catching more balls or throwing straighter, and so she builds confidence as she achieves what she aimed for.

Your 6-year-old needs lots of understanding and patience as from time to time she may be difficult and disobedient, sometimes because she is worried about something at school.

Try to help your child learn to predict how others will react to what she says or does. If your child needs it, help her with friendship skills, taking turns, playing fair, being friendly, sharing, and thinking about how others feel. And always let her know that you have confidence in her.

Six-year-olds are learning to think about values, right and wrong, fair and unfair, truth and untruth. They are likely to see values and rules from a very black-and-white viewpoint. If it is right it is right, and if it is wrong it is wrong, and there are no in-betweens. They can get quite upset about rule breaking and unfairness. They are very aware of the example you set in these areas and challenge what you do and say. They also ask lots of questions as they work out what it all means.

They may spend more time making up rules for games than they do in the actual play; this is all part of learning about rules, values and negotiation. They may also challenge your rules about things such as homework, mealtimes and bedtimes. It helps if you discuss the reasons for these rules with them and, when you can, include their ideas in setting their limits.

Badru in Year Two at school was very unhappy. The boy he really wanted to be his friend was friendly one day and rejected Badru the next. It was affecting his schoolwork and self-esteem. His parents talked with the teacher about it and she gave Badru some special responsibilities in the classroom which helped him feel valued and gave him some status with the other children. The parents talked to Badru about having different friends, not just one special one. In the holidays they made sure that he had play dates with other boys and not the one he had problems with. The next year, with new friends and support and encouragement from parents and teacher, Badru had a very happy and successful year at school.

Bullying and teasing

Making friends and belonging to a group is very important in middle childhood and onwards, and there is often unkindness and bullying as children struggle to find their place in their social world. If your child is being bullied or bullying others, and it continues, she needs help because this can be serious and long-lasting. If your child is bullying others, talk to her about how other children feel and the other ways that she could relate to them. Also think about what is happening in other parts of her life that could be causing her to be upset and angry. If she is being bullied, you could talk with her about what she could do or would like to try. For example, she could play in a different place, pretend not to notice (if it is verbal) or stay near a friend – but these things are hard for young children to do. It is important that the school knows what is happening and takes action to prevent it. If talking to the teacher about it does not make a difference, you will need to follow up until you are sure your child is safe. Most schools have anti-bullying policies and procedures to follow.

Sometimes the bullying takes the form of not being allowed to play in a particular group. You can help by listening to how your child feels and letting her know that you believe that things will get better for her. Remind her of times when she does have friends and is part of the group; this will help her build on her strengths. Having different friends over for play dates may help. Again, check with the teacher because he or she is in a good position to see what is happening and help. For many children, being left out is not ongoing. It happens from time to time for most children.

Speech and language

Six-year-olds speak clearly, using most parts of grammar in the same way as adults. They are using complex words and know thousands of words. Most have mastered difficult sounds although sometimes they may stammer getting a word out if under stress. They can tell stories, tell and enjoy jokes and riddles, and know special days and dates such as birthdays if they have been told. They can take turns in a conversation and can hold an ongoing conversation on a topic. They are able to talk about feelings, as well as about more tangible things and happenings, which is helpful for them in managing their own feelings.

Your 6-year-old no longer always needs to have pictures in the stories you read to her and she is starting to enjoy longer stories where you might read a chapter each night. She is getting to be a true reader. Instead of struggling to make sense of written words, she happily reads words and signs and reads simple stories to her baby brother or sister. Encourage her to write and illustrate her own stories, while still reading to her often. The enjoyment of reading she is learning now will last throughout her life.

Thinking and learning

Your 6-year-old can understand left and right, for example when putting on shoes, and has a good understanding of time such as yesterday, today, tomorrow and in a few days' time. Being at school gives her an interest in numbers and patterns, such as counting things she sees, thinking about the patterns of days (morning, afternoon, evening), patterns in pictures and drawings, and patterns in the way things are done (from cleaning teeth after eating and before bed, to cooking simple recipes).

She is curious about how things work and asks lots of questions to clarify situations and ideas that she does not understand. She can understand even and odd numbers.

She may be getting homework most nights and needs you to set aside 15 minutes or so of uninterrupted time when you are available for help and support if she needs it.

She is able to concentrate better than she could previously and focus on what she is doing for longer. However, she still has a relatively short attention span when learning new skills and learns best if she has changes of task and activity and some breaks in what she is doing.

Six-year-olds may also be thinking differently about death. Younger children are sad when someone they know or a special pet dies but they do not understand that it is final. They believe that the person or animal can come back. Between the ages of 6 and 7, children begin to understand that this doesn't happen and may become worried that someone who is sick might die. Your 6-year-old may ask very detailed questions as she comes to terms with new knowledge and she will be helped by explanations about the life cycles of all living things and you talking about your own beliefs. She may ask repeated questions until she really has a grasp of what she wants to know.

Problem-solving skills

It is important to help your child to learn problem-solving skills rather than just give answers or suggestions for what to do. Children gain in confidence from solving their own problems and the skills they learn will assist them in the future.

Some steps to teaching problem solving

1. Work out what the problem really is in a solvable way – sometimes this is clear e.g. when she can't find her pencils. Sometimes, however, it needs thinking through to understand it in a way that she can do something about e.g. when she has had an argument with a friend. In the case of arguing with a friend, if your child says something like 'She is just stupid', she is not thinking about the problem in a useful way. If she says 'She hates me' or 'She always wants to play a game I don't like', there are some options to consider in how to solve the problem.

2. Ask your child how it makes her feel – feelings can get in the way of problem solving if they are not in the open.

3. Ask her for her ideas about what she could do. Make a list, including even the seemingly impossible ones for consideration.

4. Talk about how the ideas would work in practice.

5. Get her to choose one that she would like to try.

6. Talk through how she is going to do it.

7. Later, check back and see if it has helped – if not try something else. (This step is important because it avoids a sense of failure.)

> **Note:** With simple problems, such as finding lost pencils you don't, of course, need to go through the whole process – just ask her to think about how she will find them.

Play

Your 6-year-old is most likely a healthy, energetic young person who enjoys active pursuits such as riding her bike or scooter, swimming and going to adventure playgrounds. She enjoys learning some ball skills with Mum or Dad or friends in the backyard and going on nature walks that include exploring and climbing. Six-year-olds also love listening and dancing to music, which is helpful for their balance and coordination as well.

Six-year-olds enjoy children's television and some cartoons and movies which are meant for older children, such as superhero movies, and may include violence. Limiting her viewing of these shows, and watching with her so you can talk about them, helps her get them into perspective. Many children of this age enjoy nature and animal programs; again it is helpful to watch with your child as some of these programs can be disturbing to children and they are real.

She is starting to get more enjoyment out of board games as she gains more skill in thinking about how to play.

Six-year-olds enjoy easy storybooks they can read for themselves and longer stories that you read to them. They may enjoy reading the same books over again as they gain confidence in recognising the words.

Most of all, your 6-year-old loves to play with friends and the complex symbolic games that they play together are important to their brain development and for learning skills such as persistence, self-control, planning, negotiation and reasoning.

Joining in play

There are some skills that children need to be able to successfully join in playing with a group. Some children just seem to learn these naturally; others sometimes need a bit of help. If your child seems to have trouble with joining in, either hanging back or pushing in and maybe getting rejected, you could watch out for these occasions and coach her with the following skills.

Joining groups skills

- Watch first and see what the group is doing.
- Go near the group and smile – look friendly.
- Say something that fits in with the game the others are playing e.g. 'That is a good train, I could collect the tickets for people who want to get on.' This often works better than just asking to play.
- Join into the game – share and take turns and cooperate.

Sleeping

Generally 6-year-olds sleep well through the night and do not need parent support unless they have worries or are unwell. Keeping to a relaxing routine before bed helps your child to calm down from the business of the day, and a time together at bedtime is a good opportunity for her to share thoughts and feelings, a practice which can last into adolescence.

Some children have nightmares as they process all that is happening in their lives and need some comforting; some still have fears of the dark or burglars or other things they have heard about. Reassurance and/or a night-light or open door often help, depending on what your child feels comfortable with.

Sexual development

Six-year-olds spend a lot of time with older children or children with older brothers and sisters and are hearing lots more about sexuality. Some ask lots of questions about subjects such as sexual intercourse or being gay that they may not have thought about before. There may also be whispering, jokes and secrets as children pick up society's attitudes to sexuality as being something you don't talk about. Answering questions honestly and simply helps children to see that this is a normal part of living and something that can be talked about. If you find it hard to start a conversation with your child, you could find a children's book about it that can open the way to talking and let her know that it is OK to talk to you. Some children may worry about masturbation, that it is bad or harmful, and need reassurance. If children masturbate a lot, or in public, it is likely to be because they have something worrying them that they need help with.

Six-year-olds are also thinking more about what it means to be a man and a woman in our society. Your child is seeing lots of different kinds of relationships in her friends' homes. For example, having friends whose parents are separating can make your child anxious about her own situation.

It is important that children feel good about whichever gender they are. This is helped by seeing parents who value their own gender as well as respect and value people, especially partners, of the other gender. Showing this to your child through what you do and what you say is important for her own wellbeing.

Emmy asked her mother, 'Which mum of Dan's mums is the mum and which one is acting as the dad?'

Her mother said, 'I don't know, they call themselves Mum 1 and Mum 2 so they are both mums – we could ask them'.

Emmy said: 'Well which mum helped make Dan because that will be the one acting as the mum'.

Her mother said, 'There are lots of different kinds of families and they do things in different ways. Some families just have one mum and some have just a dad, and some have two mums like Dan's or two dads. We can ask Dan's mums what they do in their family'.

Emmy is learning to make sense of the world. She is asking questions about a family she has known for many years but she had not previously thought about how they are different from her family. Children try to make new information fit with the things they already know about, so Emmy is trying to work out how Dan's family could fit into the way her family works and what she knows about how babies are made. She is learning that, as she gets new information, she sometimes needs to change the understanding that she had before.

Your child at school

Australia has developed an *Australian Curriculum* (www. australiancurriculum.edu.au) so that there is consistency and quality in what all Australian children learn. The aims of this national curriculum are to help children become successful learners, confident individuals and active and informed citizens. The curriculum covers the areas that will allow children to achieve this and focuses on the skills they need to learn now and in the future, as well as the content that they will learn. Lots of the teaching for young children involves hands-on play and manipulating materials, with the teacher helping them to see the patterns and meaning in what they do.

Mathematics

Here are some examples from the *Australian Curriculum* of what children will learn in Year One in Mathematics:

- learning what they can do with numbers up to 100, including counting, adding and subtracting
- understanding about things dividing into parts, such as two equal halves making a whole
- learning about Australian coins and what they mean (simple shopping tasks such as giving your child money to buy an ice-cream and working out together what coins she needs help put this into practice)
- measuring size and shapes and volume
- skip counting – counting by twos and fives and tens
- starting to learn about telling the time.

English (Language, Literature, Literacy)[31]

In Year One children have lots of practice with reading and learning about the use of words. Here are some examples from the *Australian Curriculum*:

- learn about how words make up sentences and about simple punctuation such as capital letters and full stops
- learn the different uses of writing and to think and talk about what they have read
- use language in conversation and give short presentations to their class on topics they are interested in.

Year One students also need to learn the words on their list of 'sight words'. These words are the most commonly used words in the English language and once children know these they have a good foundation for reading. They may be expected to know 50 sight words by the end of Year One. These words don't usually have a picture that goes with them, but are words that children need to recognise (e.g. from, and, with, but). Your child may get some sight words for homework; once she knows these she may be given a book to read with some of them in it.

As your 6-year-old starts to write sentences she often makes up words with her own spelling. Schools are not usually concerned about this with beginning writers as it is important for them to learn to get pleasure from being able to write their words, not to have their first efforts heavily corrected. They gradually learn to spell from reading. Of course, when you write something for them it needs to be spelt correctly.

You can help your child by reading lots of stories. Even when she can read some stories it is still very enjoyable to be read to. You can help by getting her to read simple things for you; for example, 'Would you look at the notice on the door and see if the shop is open yet?' 'What is the next thing on the list I have to buy?'

You can also help by taking an interest in the topics your 6-year-old is learning about and assisting her in following her interests. Her interests are expanding rapidly, such as what goes on in the world around her, local history, and building on discussions at school.

Some other things to know about 6- to 7-year-olds

Living skills

Six-year-olds are very independent about most aspects of living. They can dress themselves, clean their teeth, eat properly with whatever eating utensils you use and be responsible, with reminders, for some household tasks such as picking up toys, feeding pets and setting the table. Some tasks such as homework still need adult support and you taking an interest is a good way of motivating your child and showing her that you believe the task is important.

Your 6-year-old takes more interest in the world around her, both from what she learns at school and from interacting with others. One practical benefit from this is that she is probably happy to try a greater variety of foods and be interested in why different foods are important, even if she was a fussy eater when younger.

Optimism

When children begin school and experience new challenges, they may compare themselves with others and lose confidence. Helping them to learn optimism is an approach that will assist them to counteract negative self-evaluation and think positively.[32]

Optimism is a view of looking at life and what happens to you in a positive way. People who have this optimistic view of life are less likely to feel depressed and more likely to succeed and persevere at things because they believe in a good outcome. It is one of the qualities that contribute to good mental health and coping skills when things go wrong.

Optimistic people, if something goes wrong, look for a cause and a solution. Pessimistic people are more likely to think bad things always happen to them and it will never change. They look for someone to blame – often themselves.

Optimism should be grounded in reality, and look at practical issues and solutions.

Optimism is learned from the way parents and carers talk to children, and from children's experiences of persevering and achieving success.

Some of the ways that parents can help children develop an optimistic outlook include:

- Challenge pessimistic views. Help your child to re-think. Some examples appear in the table below.

Table 7.1. Challenging pessimistic views

Pessimistic view	Optimistic view
I can't.	Not yet. With practice you will.
No-one likes me.	You had no-one to play with today. Yesterday you played with your friends.
I always get it wrong.	Remember the last time you did this, and you did it well. Sometimes you get hard things wrong, but often you get them right.
It was my fault that I was late for school.	Today it took a long time to get ready. Tomorrow we can think of a way to be quicker.

- Give your child opportunities to persevere and succeed. Encourage your child with tasks that she can succeed at and give her praise for her effort and sticking at it, not just for the result.
- Think about and perhaps change your own approach to what you do and say. Young children copy and model themselves on their parents and special adults in their lives. Your self-talk and what you say to others affects how your children see the world.
- For example a pessimistic person might say: 'I'm so stupid, I've forgotten what I needed to get at the shop.' An optimistic person might say 'Oh, I've forgotten what I had to get from the shop. I had too many things to remember. Next time I will write myself a note.' Self-talk like this helps children to think optimistically.

Overview – Six to Seven

Six-year-olds are taking a big step forward into the world. Friendships become very important and there may be lots of ups and downs as children work out how to be a friend and how to cope when things go wrong. Thinking skills are growing and understanding of things like time, space, reading and using numbers is becoming easier. At the same time more is expected of your 6-year-old at school, such as regular homework. Plenty of physical exercise helps her to run off excess energy and gives some freedom after days in the classroom. As a parent of a 6-year-old, you will need patience, consistency and good humour as your child becomes more demanding in many ways as she copes with challenges of school life and developing friendships.

Remember that this is a general guide. All children develop differently depending on their own qualities and their environment. If your child is very out-of-step with other children of the same age it is important to talk it over with a health professional, in case there is a problem that needs help.

Physical development
- loses first teeth
- occasionally wets pants
- confident physical skills
- learns some new ball skills
- needs good sleep.

Social/emotional development
- friendships becoming more important
- belonging to a group is important
- compares herself with others
- usually not a good loser
- starts to challenge rules.

Speech and language

- speaks clearly and well
- reads simple texts but still needs to be read to
- enjoys holding conversations
- can talk about feelings
- likes jokes and simple riddles.

Thinking and learning

- understands left and right
- beginning to tell the time
- interested in numbers and counting
- growing attention span, but still needs changes of activity
- plays complex symbolic games
- can remember several things when asked e.g. to do an errand that has several different parts.

Toys for 6-year-olds

- computer (this is a big present but will be very useful)
- balls and bats
- books
- basketball and hoop to throw into
- appropriate DVDs
- scooter with helmet
- two-wheeled bike with helmet (and probably trainer wheels)
- swimming goggles
- kickboard
- board games
- skipping rope
- dolls, dollhouse and furniture
- LEGO®
- craft kits
- painting materials.

Chapter 8
Seven to Eight

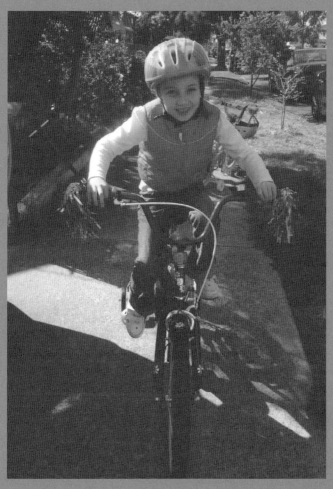

Fitness and fun

Seven-year-olds have made big steps in confidence and knowledge and are often therefore more settled and at ease than in the previous year. They have been at school for a year or more and have mostly overcome earlier difficulties with the new environment and new learning. Negotiating friendships and belonging to a group are still very important and there could be times when children believe they have no-one who likes them – this is more likely with girls than boys as many boys are starting to identify more with sports than group belonging. Seven-year-olds are likely to be good triers at whatever they do, look forward to doing well and get down in the dumps if they think they are not succeeding. They still need lots of encouragement and reassurance.

Middle childhood

The years between 6 and 12 are often called middle childhood. Children's development in thinking enables them to look at things from other people's viewpoint, to think about feelings and how they manage different situations, to wait for something they want, and to compare themselves with others. They have more understanding of differences and similarities between people such as differences in culture, in beliefs, in talents and abilities, and family customs. They are thinking about gender roles and what it means to be male or female and about their cultural identity. They are much more likely than before to be influenced by feelings such as shame and embarrassment and might try to hide a situation where they feel they have done something wrong. They are also much more aware of belonging or not belonging to the group and of prejudice and discrimination. They are developing a sense of identity – who they are and where they fit in.

> Saba says to her mother, 'I am a good singer because you are a good singer, but some people aren't good singers because their mothers aren't good singers'.
>
> *Saba is thinking about her identity and relating it to what she can do. She is also thinking about what helps to form identity although still in a very practical way, using what she sees and knows.*

Families are crucial in helping children to develop a positive sense of identity and values that will assist them to make constructive life choices. This comes from what they do as a family and from making time to talk with children and helping them to think about new situations and ideas. Every experience and interaction that happens throughout your child's day impacts on his understanding of the world and where he fits in it, as well as on his own sense of confidence, competence and wellbeing. You are still, to a large extent, the mirror in which he sees himself, although he is now being more influenced by peers and teachers.

The importance of communication

Positive communication is at the centre of helping children to learn to value themselves and others and to make sense of the world and how they fit in it. It starts with listening. Often when children ask us something, we answer with advice or information without really knowing what is behind the question or don't help them to learn to think it through for themselves. Some questions or prompts that help conversations include:

- 'That's interesting, where did you hear that?'
- 'What do you think?'

- 'Tell me more about what happened.'
- 'How did that make you feel?'
- Or even just 'Uh-huh' or 'Yes'

When your child feels really heard, you can make suggestions for him to think about or where you both might find out more. For example:

- 'I am not really sure about that, perhaps we could look it up.'
- 'Can you remember a time when you really did well at that?'
- 'What do you think would help?'

You might have to give your own opinions but helping your child to think something through helps him develop confidence in his own ability. You might also remind him that mistakes are helpful because we learn from them and that everyone makes them. You can help him to value trying and persevering as well as succeeding and to value himself and what he can do. It is your relationship with him and communication with him that supports him in finding his place in his world.

For more information about what supports healthy development in middle childhood see the Search Institute website.[33]

Physical development

Your 7-year-old is physically well-coordinated and learning the skills he will need to play team sports. It is recommended that children under 8 do not play competitive sport, but they can learn the skills such as running, swimming, bat or racquet and ball, kicking, throwing and catching balls, throwing balls into a hoop, junior gym and dancing. Many of these can be done in the backyard or park and are very good for children's physical coordination and confidence. They give children an opportunity to see which sports they enjoy and might like to play in the future.

Aside from physical fitness, there is a lot that children can learn from playing sport, such as controlling their impulses (you can't play a good shot if you lose your temper), working together in a team and managing feelings about winning and losing. The main thing is, when your child does begin playing team sport, that he enjoys it and has fun – this is what encourages him to continue playing. Therefore, it is important when you are looking for a team for your child to join in the next few years that you choose one which is not too competitive at first and where all children in the team have a chance to play and succeed.

Your 7-year-old can ride his bicycle without trainer wheels and may still also be enjoying his ability with a scooter.

Your child's better eye–hand coordination means that he can draw and paint accurately and do crafts with fairly small and intricate patterns. Some 7-year-olds enjoy making simple models such as aircraft, as well as doing constructions with LEGO®. Some may also show interest in learning how to sew and knit.

Social and emotional development

Now that they have had more than a year at school, some children can be very confident and ready to push the boundaries a bit – so there may be some rough play or excluding other children from groups.

Your 7-year-old wants to be part of a group of friends, as children need to establish a place in their group of peers in order to move forward into growing up. For children who are not invited to be in the group it can be very distressing. Children of this age should be able to understand how other children feel but may need to be reminded – they also feel vulnerable and are unsure whether they will still be in the group if they support someone who is not. If you have a child who is on the outer and feeling sad about it, talk to the teacher. Firstly, teachers have a different viewpoint and may say that your child has friends to play with most days. How your child feels is important and needs to be taken seriously; however you may be reassured after talking with the teacher. Secondly, children really admire their teachers and the teacher may well be able to help the children, including your child, re-think what they are doing and play more inclusively.

Winning and losing well is important and contributes to self-esteem. Children need to feel some confidence that they can win sometimes before they are able to cope with the disappointment of losing, so still playing games such as Snap where your child wins will help. It also helps to remind him of times he does things well and assist him to persevere with things he wants to achieve.

Children can be very competitive and need help to learn to value their own qualities rather than always comparing themselves with others.

Seven-year-olds are very interested in rules – rules of games and rules of society. They practise these by making up rules for games. Sometimes the rule-making takes on more importance than the game. Your 7-year-old is also concerned with what is fair and what is not fair. They may challenge your rules and say they are unfair, or pick up on inconsistency. These challenges are good teaching and negotiating opportunities. Also, it is worthwhile to consider what you do yourself, because children learn much from the adults they model themselves on. So, if telling the truth is a quality you value highly, you would not ask your child to tell someone on the phone or at the door that you are not at home when you are. You can however talk with your child about when telling the truth may not be helpful, for example, when they have just been given a gift that they don't like. Talking these things through and listening to your child's viewpoint helps him to work through all the values challenges that will come in the next few years. It also helps him to know that he can turn to you with problems and you will not just give advice, but listen as well.

Your 7-year-old can be very sensitive at times and lose confidence if something does not go well. Your encouragement and reassurance are important. He may have fears related to what he sees and hears in the media and he is at an age where you can discuss these with him to give him more understanding. The main fear of many children of primary school age is losing a parent or family break-up and they need lots of support if there are family problems.

In Western communities, such as Australia, 7-year-old children and older usually form their play groups according to their gender – boys play with boys and girls with girls.

Speech and language

Your 7-year-old speaks well and can take his place in conversations with you about a variety of topics. He can talk with good recall about what has happened in the past and about plans for the future and uses complex sentences and generally good grammar to do this. By the end of the year he can write a short story that is easy for adults to read. He is likely to talk to you about words and the meanings of new and complicated words that he comes across. Reading is becoming a pleasure as children become more adept at it, although being read to is a joy that usually continues for many years.

Your 7-year-old is also developing his critical listening abilities, so that he can notice, for example, when something on the media is clearly exaggerated or untrue or when others make a mistake in their speech. He can also remember more of what you tell him and follow directions which include a number of steps.

He should be able to take messages on the telephone and make phone calls to well-known numbers by the end of this year.

Thinking and learning

Seven-year-olds are keen for knowledge and want to find out about many things. Helping your child to find his own information rather than just giving an answer will give him skills for a lifetime. The internet can be a useful source of information, and skills in using the computer are valuable. You can give children a solid grounding by teaching them the basics of using the keyboard as well as explaining about the need to look at sites that are reputable. Sites that are run by governments or educational organisations are likely to have correct information and are a good place to look first.

A child's quest for information in great detail sometimes seems a bit bizarre to adults, but this is your child's way of making sense of the world.

Seven-year-olds can think in a more complex way than younger children, for example, they can hold in mind several different aspects of a group. They can look at a group of animals which may have several different kinds of animal and understand that each animal has its own name (e.g. cow) and is also part of the bigger group (animals). In their own family they can understand that there are children and adults, some who may be male and some who may be female, and all are people as well as being family members. They are able to think more logically and can sometimes go back over what they have done and see where it went wrong.

Seven-year-olds are also learning that things can be the same even though they look different. A glass of water poured into a jug still has the same amount of water or a number of blocks spread out over a bigger area still has the same number of blocks. However they are still learning this and if you offer seven year olds a choice between a dollar coin and five twenty cent coins, most will take the twenty cent coins because they look like more money.

Seven-year-olds are thinking more critically about many things and most will be starting to question how beings like Father Christmas and fairies can be real, much as they would like them to be. (One 7-year-old who was thinking about this took a very practical point of view and told her mother that she no longer believed in fairies but she did still believe in the tooth fairy.) Seven-year-olds still haven't entirely given away these beliefs but they are starting to question how they fit in with the real world that they know. If you are asked, one suggestion might be to tell your child the story of King Wenceslaus or St Nicholas and talk about how their spirit lingers on in the story of Father Christmas and giving at Christmas. Children are beginning to think about values and moral issues and giving to others is one way they could contribute. There are many charities which make up Christmas gifts for disadvantaged children which your child could contribute to.

Three-year-old Hawa asked at bedtime if she could make cakes. Her mother said, 'No, it is bedtime and all the children are going to sleep'. Her seven-year-old sister Kayla said, 'No, Mummy, on the other side of the world it is daytime and some children will be getting up and making cakes'. Their mother said, 'Well we are not on the other side of the world.' Kayla said, 'But it's still true that at this exact time some children are getting up'.

Kayla is thinking logically and also now sometimes challenges her parents, rather than thinking everything they say must be right. In the last sentence she is still looking to her mother to affirm what she says.

Your child at school

Learning expands at school in Year 2 in many different areas, such as learning about society, history and the world we live in. The following are examples from the *Australian Curriculum* of what your child might learn in Mathematics and English in Year 2.

Mathematics[34]

While technology can help in many ways the ability to use mathematical reasoning is fundamental to all areas of life, for example, driving, shopping, choosing, cooking and science. It is about collecting and analysing information, using numbers and other skills to solve problems.

Beginning mathematics is about:

- learning to be familiar with and understand numbers up to 1000
- doing simple adding up and subtraction
- measuring and comparing things of different shapes and sizes

- learning about chance and data e.g. make a graph of all the favourite colours in the class
- using a calendar and a simple map
- telling the time in five-minute intervals using digital and analogue clocks.

English (Language, Literature, Literacy)

Being able to confidently use language in every situation is one of the most important foundations for all other learning. As your child moves through Year 2 he will have many opportunities to practise with language in different ways. (By the time he is 8 he will be able to read fluently and understand what he is reading.) Here are some examples:

- continuing practice in reading
- understanding the ways words go together in sentences
- more complex ways of writing sentences and using words
- different uses of texts such as stories, guides for how-to-do things, rules and directions
- thinking about the stories he reads, asking questions about what could happen next and why, and maybe what else could happen
- writing his own ideas about the stories, and writing his own stories with a beginning, middle and end
- practice in using language for conversations and presenting ideas to others.

You can help by taking an interest in what your child is telling you about the new things he is learning at school, encouraging him with homework, helping him find information he needs, making sure he has uninterrupted time and space to do his homework, helping him to have access to a computer and supporting school activities.

> **Note:** Parents tread a fine line with homework between being encouraging and being too demanding, which can lead to discouragement. Your child needs to see that you take an interest and value homework and that it is important for him to complete it. However, together with encouragement to persevere, sometimes he needs a break, a bit of help with difficult homework, and maybe a snack before he begins doing it (if it is at the end of the school day).

Some other things to know about 7- to 8-year-olds

After-school activities

Seven-year-olds are likely to be interested in some out-of-school activities including music, dance, art, drama, crafts, gym, swimming and so on. They also need time just to play. Much of the important learning in their lives takes place in play. So, while it is good to let your child try activities to get an idea of what he likes, and also to gain some of the personal skills such as persistence that are important to his learning, it is also important to have a balance. He needs time to do homework and home chores, time to play, time to be with friends and time to just be!

Your 7-year-old might have to choose between several possible activities, perhaps choosing the one that his friends go to, or one he has a particular interest in. If, after giving an activity a good try, your child does not enjoy it, he has learned more about himself and maybe what else he might want to try later. Craft, music, art or sporting skills begun in childhood can lead to a lifetime of enjoyment, and contribute to resilience.

Values

Seven is a good age to be talking about values as children's thinking skills are developing rapidly and they are starting to think more widely and deeply about what they see and do, and how they behave in relation to others. Your 7-year-old is still more likely to want to please you than to tell the truth. If he tells you an 'untruth' about something he has done in order to please you, you could talk to him about how you value the truth – it usually works much better to use this as teaching time, rather than to punish. Most schools have values such as cooperation and caring that they explicitly teach to children. Although you will have been talking about values as they come up and living by the values that are important to you, your child is now likely to want to talk and think more about such values as:

- playing fair
- winning and losing
- telling the truth
- respecting other people's belongings
- helping a friend who is being teased or left out
- playing by the rules
- difference and disability.

Some of these issues are difficult for children because they need to be accepted by their group and it is hard for them to do something the group would not like. Talking about why values matter and how they make people feel is a good start. If you listen without judging to your child's point of view, you are opening the way for him to be able to talk to you about all sorts of worries.

Learning about certain values may be new to some children. In some families whatever they have belongs to everyone; if a child takes something he wants, it is not thought of as stealing but part of communal ownership. A child may take something he wants from another child without realising that it is not allowed in particular circumstances.

> Rose was sitting next to Abby who was a very confident student. When the group was asked to do a writing task Rose copied Abby's. Rose was very surprised when the teacher told her to do her own work. She said, 'I was copying Abby's because hers is better and I wanted to do the best I can'.
>
> *Rose had not heard of the concept of cheating and was acting on previous knowledge which was to do her best. The importance of doing one's own work individually was new learning.*

Some ways to help children think about values include:

- read stories that involve values – including fairy tales and stories about heroes and heroines from the past
- talking about your own values and how you live by them, how some things are not straightforward and there are shades of grey e.g. not always being honest if you don't like a gift
- encourage and show approval for children who make thoughtful, value-based choices.

Overview – Seven to Eight

Seven-year-olds have many of the qualities they need for independence. They are physically well-coordinated, have most of the everyday living skills they need and have much more ability to reason and remember than they had a year ago. Your 7-year-old is able to understand what is real and what is not real, although the remains of magical thinking are still there as he takes care not to step on a crack in the footpath. He is very much part of his group of playmates and seeks to be in activities or clubs with them. His confidence is still easily broken and he needs parent support even though he sometimes now challenges you. All children are different and the information below is a general guide about what you might expect. If you have concerns about your child talk with a teacher or health professional.

Physical development

- physically well-coordinated
- can learn sporting skills
- rides bicycle without trainer wheels
- good eye–hand coordination: can draw and paint accurately and do crafts with fairly small and intricate patterns, may learn to knit or sew
- makes simple models such as aircraft.

Social/emotional development

- wants to be part of a group of friends
- usually forms groups according to gender
- winning and losing is important and contributes to self-esteem
- very interested in rules and fairness
- can be competitive
- can be sensitive and needs encouragement

- takes responsibility
- shows care and concern for others.

Speech and language
- speaks well and can take his place in conversations
- speech should be easy to understand for people who don't know him
- can write a short story that is easy for adults to read
- reading is becoming a pleasure
- takes messages on the telephone and makes phone calls to well-known numbers.

Thinking and learning
- looks for knowledge and likes finding out things
- can hold more things in mind
- good recall about the past
- able to plan
- able to see things from another's point of view

Toys for 7-year-olds
- bicycle and bicycle accessories
- sporting equipment according to interests
- craft and music equipment according to interests
- lessons in an activity he enjoys
- books
- jigsaw puzzles
- computer
- clock
- watch
- swimming accessories – goggles, beach towel
- dolls and dollhouse
- pencils, paint and drawing books.

Chapter 9

Eight years old

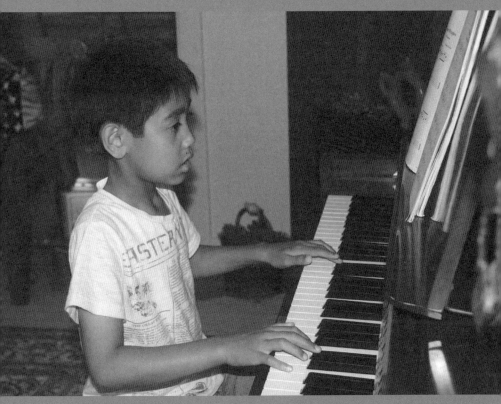

Skills for life

By now your 8-year-old child is into middle childhood and she will not be undergoing the major developmental changes that she has been through in the early years, but consolidating her learning and abilities as she moves towards puberty. Eight-year-olds who have had good opportunities to socialise and good support in the early years will have developed lots of self-confidence and are likely to be enthusiastic and outgoing. During the next three or four years they will be learning much more about the world they live in and thinking more about what they value, believe in and enjoy. Friendships with other children become still more important and they may want to belong to a particular group or club. As your child sees more of other families and ways of doing things, she may question or even challenge some of the things that you do in your home. This is a positive opportunity to discuss with her why you think as you do, why others may do things differently and most importantly to listen to her point of view as she starts to think about the things that will matter in her own future.

Physical development

The skills that your 8-year-old has been practising in the previous years – running, ball play, climbing, jumping – now come into their own. Many 8-year-olds want to join junior teams and try out the sports they enjoy. This can be a good start to continuing to play a sport as they grow up. Check out the team first, and try to find one where the coach is not too competitive. At this age all children in a team need to be given an opportunity to play and enjoy learning the game and the rules about fair play, winning and losing. Learning to be a member of a team, taking turns, sharing with others, playing fair, obeying the coach, being a 'good sport' and getting exercise are what it is about when first starting team sports. It will encourage your child if you take an interest, watching the games, encouraging and helping out when parents are needed. Continuing to practise ball skills with her at home or in the park if she wants to is another way to help her enjoy the activities.

Children who decide they are not athletic, or don't enjoy the games, still need some physical exercise so may need help exploring other options that don't involve teams, such as bicycle riding, walking the dog, gardening or swimming.

Your child's fine motor skills are good and she can do more intricate work with model making or building complex LEGO® constructions and other craft work, as well as draw and paint well with lots of detail. She also has more finger control for learning to play an instrument.

Social and emotional development

Eight-year-olds are very committed to their friendship groups, teams, friends and often a best friend. It is knowing they can be a good friend and have friends that helps them to gradually move away from dependence on family as they grow into adolescence.

Since friends are so important, there can be times when children will try to exclude another child to try to keep their own place in the group, or break up a best friendship because they want to be friends with someone else. This can be very hurtful as all children need to know they are liked and included in their group. Most children have times when they are upset about friendships, especially girls – boys often get more status from sport. If it happens on the odd occasion you can support your child by encouraging her to find someone else to play with, maybe have a new friend over and, of course, by asking and supporting what she would like to do. Maybe she just wants you to listen! You can also remind her of all the times that other children have wanted to play with her. If it seems to happen often, or your child is very distressed, the next step would be to talk with the teacher about it. If the teacher is not able to help, talk with a health professional about it because ongoing unhappiness damages children's confidence and wellbeing.

Your 8-year-old is capable and confident in what she can do and likes to solve her own problems, but she can be very sensitive to criticism and needs lots of affirmation from you. Even though she may question what you do and think as she compares this with what she knows of the world, she still really needs parents' love, support and belief. She needs you to be there to listen and understand and help her to think through her problems.

Peer influence is strong and it is important to your child that she does the same things and has the same things as others in her group in order to feel that she really belongs. If she wants to do or have something that you are unsure of, check with other parents. It may seem to her that 'everyone' has something she wants, when in reality it is only one or two other children. Sometimes she will want something that is clearly inappropriate for her age, for example, a mobile phone. Apart from the risk of losing them, mobile phones can mean access to inappropriate or harmful messages. Of course, it is very important for parents to know where children are, but not to rely on locating them through a mobile phone at this age.

She now enjoys sleepovers with friends and on school trips. If your child still wets the bed (and a few 8-year-olds will for the next year or two), and there is an overnight school trip coming up, remember to let the teacher know. You can reassure your child that the school knows how to deal with this without letting other children know.

Eight-year-olds still have some fears including losing a parent, not being liked, the dark, snakes and burglars.

> Jed was going to the shop with his dad. His dad went back to get his wallet, phone and sunglasses. Jed then asked his dad to wait a minute and he went back for his own wallet and sunglasses.
>
> *Eight-year-olds identify with the same sex parent and practise the adult role as Jed practised doing the same as his father.*

Speech and language

Your 8-year-old can speak well with correct grammar, using complex sentences and ideas. She should not have difficulty with any of the speech sounds. She enjoys reading for pleasure; she also reads signs and reads and interprets directions, for example, how to do an activity. She writes simple stories and messages. She speaks well on the phone. She understands about time and talks accurately about events that have happened in the past or when things are going to happen, such as when school holidays will be.

She likes to know the reasons for things and have conversations about why and how things happen. Encourage her in these conversations; listen and take an interest in her ideas to support her in thinking more about what she wants to say. You can help her language by making sure she has books that are at her reading level and relate to her interests. Some children like to read non-fiction books about their interests.

Thinking and learning

Your 8-year-old has a growing understanding of the world around her and how she fits in it. She thinks about values such as right and wrong and fair and unfair and wants to explore these ideas with you. She may be especially upset if things happen that she sees as wrong or unfair, but is more open to looking at different viewpoints and seeing that what seems unfair to one person might seem fair to another.

She understands what is real and what is not real and no longer believes in Father Christmas or fairies.

She is a creative thinker and many 8-year-olds enjoy taking part in drama as well as other creative activities such as dance and music.

Your child has the ability to hold in mind several things at once. This enables her to do more complicated tasks and to make plans, taking into account different aspects of what will happen. For example, when planning an outing, she can think about the weather, transport, what to bring, food, clothing and so on. She can talk about how she feels, what she thinks and what she is doing.

She has by now developed some important thinking skills that will contribute to her success at school, and help her in making choices and coping with new or difficult situations. Sometimes these skills are called 'executive function' – managing yourself to be able to do what you want to.

- planning skills – thinking about something she wants to do, working out how she will do it, what she will need to make it work and predicting what might happen

- attention skills – being able to concentrate on what she is doing or what the teacher is saying without being distracted and being able to persevere or stick at something she needs to do
- flexibility – being flexible enough to change something that is not working
- emotional regulation – managing her feelings so they help her make good relationships and don't prevent her achieving what she wants to do e.g. not throw tantrums or give up, get too distressed to try
- managing behaviour – she needs to be able to stop and think before she acts and not just act on impulse: what will an action mean and what effect will it have? Playing games helps with this, including some computer games, as well as helpful feedback if she acts impulsively with friends
- working memory – being able to hold several things in her mind and use them in making plans and decisions
- evaluating and thinking about what she has done and learning from it.

If your child has problems in any of these areas you can help her by taking things slowly and helping her to organise her time and work. If she has ongoing problems in one of the areas, talk to her teacher about getting extra help.

A mother's story

When she was 7, Meg needed a costume for the end-of-school production. We went off to buy one. The shop had two options – a Christmas fairy and an elf. The fairy was pretty but a size 5 and a bit itchy due to the material. It just fitted. The elf was great and much larger. I explained that the fairy costume would only last one year and the elf was much more comfortable and would last a couple. It was a big decision but she picked the fairy. She wore it and loved it – but it did itch and she was annoyed by it.

We were cleaning up the dress-up drawer this Christmas – Meg is now 8. We found the Christmas fairy costume which is now too small to wear. I said, 'We can give that one away since you can't wear it again'. And Meg said, 'No, please I need to keep it to remind me of my bad choice'.

Meg was allowed to make a choice and has seen the consequence of her choice. Now, at 8, she has skills to evaluate choices she has made and look back and see where she has made a mistake.

Play

Eight-year-olds are beginning a transition between childhood and adolescence and their play reflects this. They still like to play with the same toys they did when they were younger, such as dolls, trucks and LEGO®, but they are also becoming interested in popular music and socialising. Many are taking up hobbies or activities related to their interests including sports, sewing, art, dance, playing an instrument or model making. Some 8-year-olds start to make collections of things that interest them, such as stamps, dolls, model cars, shells or cards. Some join a group such as Junior Lifeguard clubs. They like to play games with rules and experiment with making up rules for games. Many also enjoy puzzles, card games and board games. Your 8-year-old enjoys TV and DVDs but still needs a parent to supervise so the choice of programs is not too violent or adult in content. Watching with her and discussing the content is a good way to help her keep it in context.

Your child is probably very confident with computers and exploring what she can do with them. Check the guidelines for parents in The Digital Parent.[35] It would be a good time to make some rules about computer use, for example that computers are to be used in living rooms where everyone is, not in private places such as a bedroom. This will help to protect your child from any exploitation or abuse later on.

Sexual development

Eight-year-olds have heard a lot about sexuality but may still be unclear about some things. They have learned that it is not something people talk about and that it is often part of swearing and impolite jokes. This might mean that they don't ask you what they would like to know and some of the talk and finding out goes underground. As with younger children, if you feel that it is hard to start a conversation, showing your 8-year-old a book about the facts of life which is written for her age group will let her know that you are open to talk about it and answer questions. She should know the names of all her body parts and that she should not let anyone touch her in private parts or do anything she feels uncomfortable about. Some children of this age start to demand their own privacy in the bathroom. Keeping communication open with your child, so she can tell you if anything worries her, is important.

Your child at school

Your child is likely to be going into Year 3 during this year. Once children are in Year 3, schools are focusing on teaching the subjects in the curriculum in more formal ways and it can seem like a big step up for students from the earlier years. It is also a big step up in confidence as they can think more logically, reason things out and are really interested in understanding why things happen.

At school your child will be learning more about different subjects such as science and history and there is a lot of emphasis on the important skills of literacy and mathematics which relate to all subjects.[36]

English

At school, your 8-year-old is learning more about grammar and the parts of speech, and using language in many different ways. She explores different points of view in the books she reads. She can talk and write about different aspects of the story and what aspects of stories she likes and why. She can plan and present short talks to her class. She can take an active part in discussions, presenting her own viewpoint and appropriately questioning others. She can put what she writes and presents in a sensible order, using correct grammar and punctuation. Fluency with language and enjoyment of reading underpin almost everything she needs to do now and in the future. Her learning is still very hands-on and she learns much through seeing and doing.

Mathematics

Here are some examples of what your child might be learning about in mathematics. She now knows numbers up to 10 000 and is learning multiplication and division as well as adding, subtraction and measurement. She does more complex work with data and graphing, for example, counting the children in the class and working out whether there are more boys or girls. She can work out change when shopping and understands more about money, such as how families earn money and how cards can be used to represent money. Children learn to tell the time to the nearest minute and draw simple grid maps. They do simple experiments classifying data and learn how to use mathematical skills such as addition and subtraction to solve practical problems.

Science

In science, children are conducting experiments to find out about their world and how it works. They learn about using measurements and predict what will happen when they try an experiment. They can use diagrams and simple charts to show what they have found. They are learning both about the earth and about living things and how to organise and classify what they are learning.

History

In history, your child is moving from learning about her local community to understanding the wider community that she lives in, how our community began, and about what happened in the past and how that impacts on the present. She will also learn how to find information and how different groups have contributed to our community.

National Testing

In Year 3 all children in Australia are assessed on reading, writing, language and numeracy. This is not a pass or fail test but a way for the government, parents and schools to learn more about how children are doing and where more help may be needed. It is not about what children know so much as how they are going in developing the skills they need in these areas. Schools help children to understand how the test works so they are not worried or confused about it. Parents receive a report on how their child is going and can discuss it with the school if they need to. For more information see the National Assessment Program – Literacy and Numeracy website.[37]

Some other things to know about 8-year-olds

Motivation

Parents are often concerned about children's motivation – the concern might be about your child's motivation for school or homework, practice at learning an instrument, or for keeping her room tidy. Motivation is what helps us to want to do some things and not others. There is no magic answer to motivation – children will be well-motivated to do things they really like doing and less well-motivated to do things they don't see the reason for (just as we all are).

Some things that help motivation are:

- showing real interest in what she is doing
- fostering curiosity – wondering about how to do something or what will happen can spark interest
- doing something together rather than alone
- praise for effort and perseverance and having another go if things go wrong. Praise works best if it is genuine; a child of this age quickly picks up on praise that says something is wonderful when she knows she has not made an effort. This devalues your praise and does not help motivation
- where possible relate a task to your child's interests; for example, when doing a maths problem try to make it up around something she is interested in
- success – taking on something and doing well at it.

Some things that are meant to motivate but don't work very well are:

- rewards, such as a prize. These might work for a while but do not motivate your child to do the task, only to get a reward

- comparisons with others. This tends to make a child feel inadequate or resentful
- threats of punishment or bad outcomes – 'You will never be any good, if you don't work at this.' These tend to discourage rather than encourage children.

Motivation to try and persevere is important because persistence has more impact on success than intelligence or ability.

Discipline

Your child is old enough to reason with and is interested in right and wrong. She can be included in family discussions about setting limits and boundaries as well as consequences for broken rules. Consequences, where they are needed, work best if they are short (too long and the child gives up trying) and relevant to what has gone wrong. For example, if your child plays too long and does not get her chores done, the consequence might be that the next day she has to do the chores before she plays. Consequences that are logical make sense to children, even if they don't like them. Mistakes are to learn from and giving another chance after the consequence is part of your child's learning.

If you are having discipline problems with your 8-year-old here are some possible things to try.

- Are you being fair and reasonable in your expectations of your child's abilities and time? If you are not sure, check what parents of other children in her class are expecting.
- Is your relationship with your 8-year-old going well? Sometimes busy parents with busy children can neglect taking care of their relationships but this is important. If your relationship is not going well it is worth spending some time reconnecting before working on the discipline problem. Make some unpressured

time to spend together every day doing something your child enjoys.

- Spend some time chatting at bedtime. If there is something wrong she will probably tell you, as long as you don't ask too many questions.
- Check that everything is OK at school. Stress resulting from school – friends, schoolwork or perhaps bullying – can be expressed through behaviour.
- Does your child need help with something?
- Is something going wrong at home? Some things that really worry children are family disruption, a sick parent or parents arguing a lot with each other.
- If your child is really stressed about something you may need to lower your expectations for a while, but still keep to your daily routines because these provide a sense of security.
- Think about what time of day/week the problems happen. What has been happening before and what happens after?
- Is your child's life too programmed, so there is not much freedom of choice or time to just play and be with friends?

Trying to work out, talk about and take action regarding any of the above possibilities is time well-invested in solving discipline problems. If you can't work it out, try discussing it with a close friend, relative or teacher. Often other people can see the problem more clearly than you because they are not involved.

Let your child know that you are there for her and you love her and will help her through whatever her problem is. There will always be some ups and downs in parenting. No relationship is perfect. What really matters is to make sure to reconnect and repair your relationship after any upset. Children often cannot make the first move, but will respond if you open the way without blame or criticism.

Pocket money and chores

This a good time to start pocket money if that is what you would like to do, as children have some understanding of the meaning of money. The advantage of this is that it begins to teach your 8-year-old how to manage money. How much you give her depends on what she is going to use it for and, to a certain extent, on what other children of her age are receiving, as well as what you can afford of course. If her pocket money is just for spending you would give her less than if she is expected to save some or buy particular things, such as her lunch one day a week. Different ways of looking at pocket money include just for spending; some for spending and some for saving for something she wants; some for spending and some for buying something they need such as lunch; or some for spending and some for putting away in the bank until they are older. Parents may also believe that some pocket money should be given to a charity chosen by their child (for example, one that comes to the door or a collection box in a shop). These are different ways that you could consider for your child.

The other consideration is whether children should do chores for pocket money. Some parents ask children to do specific chores for their pocket money. Some parents give children pocket money as a family member, unrelated to chores. However they might also expect children to do some chores as their contribution to the family. Other parents give pocket money and allow the child to earn a bit extra by doing specific chores.

Some things that your 8-year-old could do include:

- set the table
- empty the dishwasher
- feed pets

- put away washing
- clean inside the car
- pick up rubbish in the yard
- tidy their rooms.

Any of the above could be your 8-year-old's general, regular chores or ones she does to earn a bit of extra money. Sometimes the chores for earning extra money are not regular tasks but things that come up on occasion that someone needs help with, for example, help in the garden one day when there is planting or weeding to be done.

Overview – Eight years old

Eight-year-olds are industrious and independent. Your 8-year-old can do most things for herself. She is interested in the world around her, working out right and wrong, playing games with rules and watching what other children and adults do. She is looking for more in-depth explanations on all sorts of subjects – from the world and nature, to machines, to birth and illness and death. She may be critical in a questioning way of what parents and other children do, and also often critical of herself and worry when she makes mistakes. In spite of all her questions, she still looks up to you as her role model and for continued love and support.

Physical development
- physically well-coordinated with increasing stamina
- may start to play team games
- good fine motor skills and hand control for detailed work
- independent with daily tasks and self care.

Social/emotional development
- confident but vulnerable to criticism
- friends are very important
- belongs to groups
- may have a best friend
- some fears.

Speech and language
- clear speech – no errors with sounds
- good grammar
- can hold an ongoing conversation with an adult
- enjoys talking with friends
- asks for lots of detail about subjects they are interested in.

Thinking and learning

- no longer believes in fairies
- can hold several things in mind at once
- has problem-solving and reasoning skills
- can work some sums out in her head without using fingers
- starting to learn to multiply
- enjoys reading to herself.

Toys for 8-year-olds

Many of these will need to relate to the child's interests.

- sporting equipment
- books
- art materials – paints, sketchbooks, coloured pencils
- craft materials
- DVDs and CDs
- watch or alarm clock
- stationery
- electric train set
- dolls and dollhouse furniture
- computer games
- model-making kits
- board games
- remote-control toys
- science kits
- bike accessories
- radio
- watch.

Conclusion

Looking back over this book, it is impossible not to be impressed by the development and learning that takes place during the early years, and by what children can do and achieve. I have repeated over and over in different ways that children need their parents' support, encouragement and enjoyment. This is really the central message of this book. As parents, we need to know about children's development so we can have realistic expectations of our children and get ideas about how to support, nurture and guide them. They need us to love them and believe in them and have fun with them. Children have a great desire to learn and grow and explore the world, and with parental love and support they will move forward confidently into middle childhood, adolescence and their future.

If you would like to know more

Your child from birth to eight is not an academic text. It is a practical book which covers general development and many of the questions/issues that concern parents and carers. It is mostly based on research about how children learn and develop, interspersed with some practical ideas from the many parents and early childhood professionals that I have worked with. There may be topics in the book that you want to know more about and, following the References list, there are further reading recommendations provided.

The suggested books are not always the most recent but they have information about young children and parenting that is really helpful and evergreen. They are divided roughly by ages; a list of titles covering the different ages of early childhood appears at the beginning.

Some recommended websites are included as well. Many parents will be doing their own research using the internet. When you are using the internet it is wise to check that the website you are looking at has authors who are known to be knowledgeable in their area. Generally government, university or medical organisation sites are likely to be reliable. It is important to take the time to check this as anyone can put up a website and much information on the web is misleading and sometimes even dangerous. In addition, some sites have a particular viewpoint that they support. If you look at the 'About Us' section of a website it should help you get a clearer understanding of the site's purpose and its level of authority.

References

1 Australia: Ministerial Council for Education, Early Childhood Development and Youth Affairs (2010) *Engaging families in the early childhood development story. Neuroscience and early childhood development: Summary of selected literature and key messages for parenting*, Carlton Sth, VIC: MCEECDYA.

   Note: the full paper is available on the internet from <http://www.mceetya.edu.au/verve/_resources/ECD_Story-Neuroscience_and_early_childhood_dev.pdf> and is very interesting and useful.

2 UNESCO (2011) Early childhood care and education, Paris, viewed 30 November 2011, <http://www.unesco.org/new/en/education/themes/strengthening-education-systems/early-childhood/>.

3 Pringle, MK (1974) *The needs of children*, London: Hutchinson.

4 Brazelton, TB & Greenspan, SI (2000) *The irreducible needs of children: What every child must have to grow, learn and flourish*, New York: Perseus.

5 NCAST (undated) *Baby cues: a child's first language*, Seattle:NCAST.

   The set, comprising DVD and cards, is available from ACER.

6 Best, C (2002) 'Revealing the mother tongue's nurturing effects on the infant ear', *Infant Behavior & Development*, vol. 25, pp. 134–139.

   There has been a lot of research in this area. This article focuses on the work that initiated the ongoing research.

7 Acredolo, L, Goodwyn, S & Abrams, D (2011) *Baby signs: How to talk to your baby before your baby can talk*, 3rd edn, Sydney: McGraw-Hill.

8 Siegel, D (1999) *The developing mind: How relationships and the brain interact to shape who we are*, NY: Guilford.

9 Shore, R (1997) *Rethinking the brain: New insights into early development*, NY: Families and Work Institute.

10 Mcleod, S (2010) Sensorimotor stage, Simply Psychology, UK, viewed 29 November 2011, <http://www.simplypsychology.org/sensorimotor.html>.

   This website gives a simple explanation with a short video clip about the concept of object permanence.

11 Bowlby, J (2005) *A secure base: Clinical applications of attachment theory*, Abingdon, Oxon, UK: Routledge.

12 Bowlby, J (2005) *A secure base: Clinical applications of attachment theory*, (p. 31) Abingdon, Oxon, UK: Routledge.

13 Circle of Security®: Early intervention program for parents and children, US, viewed 29 November 2011, <www.circleofsecurity.net>.

14 Vanderijt, H & Plooij, F (2003) *The wonder weeks*. Arnhem, Netherlands: Kiddy World Promotions BV.

15 D'Onofrio, BM (2011) 'Consequences of Separation/Divorce for Children' in Encyclopedia on Early Childhood Development, <www.child-encyclopedia.com>

16 Gunnar, M. How young children manage stress: Looking for links between temperament and experience, US, viewed 29 November 2011, <http://www.research.umn.edu/spotlight/gunnar.html>.

17 De Schipper, JC, Tavecchio, LWC, & Van IJzendoorn, MH (2008) Children's attachment relationships with day care caregivers: Associations with positive care giving and the child's temperament. *Social Development,* vol. 17, no. 3, pp. 454–470.

18 Zero to Three (2004) Temperament in early childhood: A primer for the perplexed, viewed 29 November 2011, <http://main.zerotothree.org/site/DocServer/vol24-4a.pdf?docID=1761&AddInterest=1158>.

19 Sefton-Green, J (2004) Literature review in informal learning with technology outside school Report 7, *Futurelab Series* (pp. 1–39). Bristol: Futurelab.

20 Grotberg, EH (1995) A guide to promoting resilience in children: Strengthening the human spirit, viewed 1 December 2011, <http://resilnet.uiuc.edu/library/grotb95b.html>.

21 Luthar, SS (2006) 'Resilience in development: A synthesis of research across five decades'. In D Cicchetti and D Cohen (Eds.) *Developmental psychopathology: Risk, disorder, and adaptation* (2nd edn, vol. 3, pp. 739–795), New York: Wiley.

22 Garmezy, N (1993) 'Children in poverty: Resilience despite risk'. *Psychiatry,* 56, pp. 127–136.

23 Werner, EE (1990) 'Protective factors and individual resilience'. In SJ Meisels and JP Shonkoff (Eds.) *Handbook of early childhood intervention,* (pp. 97–116), Cambridge: Cambridge University Press.

24 Milteer, RM, Ginsburg KR & Council on Communications and Media Committee on Psychosocial Aspects of Child and Family Health (2012), The importance of play in promoting healthy child development and maintaining strong parent–child bond: Focus on children in poverty, viewed 1 February 2012, <http://pediatrics.aappublications.org/content/early/2011/12/21/peds.2011-2953>.

25 Almon, J & Miller, E (2011) The crisis in early education: A research-based case for more play and less pressure, viewed 20 January 2012, <www.allianceforchildhood.org>.

Bodrova, E & Leong, DJ (2005) Uniquely preschool: What research tells us about the ways young children learn, *Educational Leadership,* vol. 63, no. 1, pp. 44–47.

Shipley, D (2008) *Empowering children. Play based curriculum for lifelong learning* (4th edn). US: Nelson Education.

Siraj-Blatchford, I (2008) Understanding the relationship between curriculum, pedagogy and progression in learning in early childhood, *Hong Kong Journal of Early Childhood,* vol. 7, no. 2, pp. 6–13.

26 Kennedy, A & Barblett, L (2010) *Learning and teaching through play: Supporting the Early Years Learning Framework,* Deakin West, ACT: Early Childhood Australia.

27 Turner-Cobb, JA, Rixon, L & Jessop, DS (2008) A prospective study of diurnal cortisol responses to the social experience of school transition in four-year-old children: Anticipation, exposure, and adaptation, *Developmental Psychobiology,* vol. 50, no. 4, pp. 377–389.

28 Penn, A (1993) *The kissing hand.* Washington DC: Child Welfare League of America.

29 US Department of Education (2000) A call to commitment: Fathers' involvement in children's learning, viewed 12 December 2011, <http://www2. ed.gov/pubs/parents/calltocommit/chap1.html>.

30 Garth, M (1991) *Starbright: Meditations for young children.* Melbourne: Collins Dove.

31 Australian Curriculum Assessment and Reporting Authority, English, viewed 12 December 2011, <http://www.australiancurriculum.edu.au/English/ GuidedTour>.

32 Sara, H (2009) *Optimistic children: Pathways to confidence and wellbeing,* ACT, Early Childhood Australia.

33 Search Institute (2011) 40 Developmental assets for middle childhood, viewed 12 December 2011, <http://www.search-institute.org/40-developmental- asset-middle-childhood-8-12>.

34 Australian Curriculum Assessment and Reporting Authority, Mathematics, viewed 12 December 2011, <http://www.australiancurriculum.edu.au/ Mathematics/GuidedTour>.

35 The Digital Parent, viewed 12 December 2011, <http://www.thedigitalparent. com/>.

36 Australian Curriculum Assessment and Reporting Authority, Year 3, viewed 12 December 2011, <http://www.australiancurriculum.edu.au/Year3>.

37 Australian Curriculum Assessment and Reporting Authority, NAPLAN, viewed 12 December 2011, <http://www.nap.edu.au/NAPLAN/index.html>.

Early childhood resources

Bower, L (2008) *Everyday learning about imagination*, ACT: Early Childhood Australia.

Crary, E (1993) *Without spanking or spoiling*, 2nd ed, NY: Parenting Press.
This book covers a wide age range and has a section on time out which is not appropriate for toddlers; however there are many useful ideas about discipline in the book.

Faber, A & Mazlish, E (1998) *Siblings without rivalry*, NY: HarperCollins.
A very helpful book about getting along with brothers and sisters.

Faber, A & Mazlish, E (1999) *How to talk so kids will listen and listen so kids will talk*, NY: HarperCollins.

Garth, M (1991) *Starbright: Meditations for young children*, Melbourne: Collins Dove.

Grotberg, EH (1998) *A guide to promoting resilience in children: Strengthening the human spirit*, The International Resilience Project from the Early Childhood Development: Practise and Reflections series, Bernard Van Leer Foundation http://resilnet.uiuc.edu/library/grotb95b.html
You can download the above book from the internet for free, and it has excellent information about helping young children build resilience.

Hall, J (1993) *Confident kids: Helping your child cope with fear*, Port Melbourne, Vic: Lothian.

Harris, B (2005) *When your kids press your buttons and what you can do about it* London: Piatkus.
This book assists parents to work out why it is that some things your children do really seem to get to you, and what you can do about it.

Kurcinka, MS (2005) *Kids, parents and power struggles*, NY: HarperCollins.

Kurcinka, MS (2006) *Raising your spirited child: A guide for parents whose child is more intense, sensitive, perceptive, persistent, and energetic,* Rev. ed, Sydney: HarperCollins.

Linke, P (2010) *Everyday learning about managing change,* ACT: Early Childhood Australia.

Mackey, G (2006) *Everyday learning about brothers and sisters,* ACT: Early Childhood Australia.

Marston, S (1990) *The magic of encouragement: Nurturing your child's self-esteem,* William Morrow & Co.
   Available online at <http://www.stephaniemarston.com/product_details. aspx?pd=5>.

Weininger, O (2002). *Time-in parenting: How to teach children emotional self-control, life skills and problem solving,* Toronto, Canada: Caversham Publishers.
   May be difficult to obtain but is well worth the effort.

Websites about early childhood

www.aaimhi.org.au
   Australian Association for Infant Mental Health – includes papers on sleep, touch, time out and parenting after separation.

www.circleofsecurity.org
   Circle of Security – especially about attachment, early relationships and time out

http://www.mhcs.health.nsw.gov.au/topics/Early_Childhood.html
   NSW Multicultural Health Communication Service – information for parents on a wide range of health and parenting issues

www.zerotothree.org
   Zero to Three – Early childhood development with an emphasis on mental health

http://parents.vodafone.com/
   Information for parents about children and the internet.

Babies

Acredolo, L, Goodwyn, S & Abrams, D (2011) *Baby signs: How to talk to your baby before your baby can talk*, 3rd ed. Sydney: McGraw-Hill.

Gethin, A & MacGregor, B (2007) *Helping your baby to sleep*, Sydney: Finch.

Murray, L & Andrews, L (edited by Sue Parish) (2001) *Your social baby*, Camberwell, Vic: ACER.

NCAST Programs (2011) *Your baby and you: Attachment in the first year: DVD for parents and guide for professionals*. Seattle, WA: University of Washington.
    Available in Australia from ACER.

Sears, W & Sears, M (2003) *The baby book: Everything you need to know about your baby – from birth to age two*. New York: Little, Brown and Company.

Toddlers

Note: Some books about toddlers talk about the toddler years as a time of battles to be won. Toddlers learn best where parents' approach is to help them with their learning, feelings and behaviour, rather than to take an oppositional point of view.

Lieberman, A (1993) *The emotional life of the toddler*, NY: The Free Press.
    This is a very wise book about toddlers and a very good basis for understanding them.

Manolson, A et al (1995) *You make the difference: In helping your child learn*. Toronto: Hanen Centre.
    A book for parents of babies and toddlers.

Website

www.cyh.com
    Information about toilet training.

Preschool and upwards

Connor, J & Linke, P (2010) *Your child's first year at school*, Rev. ed, ACT: Early Childhood Australia.

Websites for preschool children

Note: These sites are for children and parents to use.

http://www.nickjr.co.uk/

http://www.nickjr.com

http://treehousetv.com/

http://www.disneyjunior.ca/en/

http://www.fisher-price.com/fp.aspx?st=2601&e=gamesByAge&mcat=game_infant&site=us

Websites for school beginners and upwards

Note: These sites are free and have fun activities that support what children learn at school. Some sites also have games for younger children. (Children may need some help from parents to get started.)

www.ictgames.com

www.starfall.com

www.studyladder.com

www.mathletics.com.au

www.spellingcity.com

Other helpful resources for further reading

Aarts, M (2008) *Marte Meo: Basic manual*, 2nd ed, Marte Meo International. Available from <http://www.martemeo.com/EN/webshop/marte-meo-basic-manual>.

Harvard University, Center on the Developing Child, <http://developingchild.harvard.edu>.

Seligman, ME (1995) *The optimistic child*, Sydney: Random House.

Siegel, D (1999) *The developing mind: How relationships and the brain interact to shape who we are*. NY: Guilford.

Shore, R (1997) *Rethinking the brain: New insights into early development*, New York: Families and Work Institute.